"*For William Ward, everything comes to being a fully present journey: premonitions, epiphanies, past history coming around again, moments of high hilarity, and deep, quiet, pure thankfulness for all of life—not only for what it has brought him, but for the unknowns it's cooking up right now . . . he shows how one can travel lightly in the light.*"

—CLAIRE BLATCHFORD, author, *Turning* and *Experiences with the Dying and the Dead*

"*Among the many personal accounts of the cancer experience that have been published, I have read none more honestly revealing or more beautiful than William Ward's* Traveling Light. *To read his compelling and poetic account is to meet someone you would want to know and spend serious time with. Ward's charm is not conventional; he makes no effort to captivate. He is simply an appealing, candid, accomplished person whose journal of navigation through the experience of serious cancer is a rare story of love, a unique kind of faith, and a reverence for the committed life. Even if Ward were not dealing with cancer, he would be clearly one of the most companionable, genuine human beings you would ever encounter.*"

—RICHARD GROSSMAN, psychotherapist; author, *The Tao of Emerson;* founder of the Cancer Support Program at Wainwright House, Rye, NY; former director of The Center for Health in Medicine at Montefiore Medical Center in New York; and currently Retreat Group Leader, Cancer Help Program at Smith Farm Center for Healing and the Arts, Washington, DC

TRAVELING LIGHT

walking the cancer path

❧

WILLIAM WARD

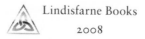
Lindisfarne Books

2008

Lindisfarne Books

PO BOX 749, GREAT BARRINGTON, MA 01230

www.lindisfarne.org

COVER IMAGE BY CLAIRE WARD MIESMER
COVER AND BOOK DESIGN: WILLIAM JENS JENSEN

LIBRARY OF CONGRESS CATALOGING-IN-PUBLICATION DATA

Ward, William, 1946–
    Traveling light : walking the cancer path / William Ward.
        p. cm.
    ISBN 978-1-58420-061-1 (alk. paper)
    1. Ward, William, 1946 — Health. 2. Brain—Cancer—
Patients—United States—Biography. I. Title.
    RC280.B7W37 2008
    362.196'994810092—dc22
    [B]
                                            2008001894

Printed in the United States of America

To my dear Andy,
You are my angel through happiness and sorrow,
through my darkest night and day clear light.
You are the joy of my life, my loving wife, my strength,
my trusted friend, my compass and my anchor.
Mother, companion, wise woman, healer, comforter.

❧

Thank you dear family and friends for helping me through this
birth. Thank you Snow White and Rose Red, my dear daughters.

❧

This book has been made possible by the work of many hands.
I especially want to thank Janet Elsbach for her friendship
and tireless editing. Thanks to our team of friends at
SteinerBooks, who made straight the way:
Christopher Bamford, Gene Gollogly,
Marsha Post, William Jensen, Mary Giddens,
and thank you Claire Blatchford for your loving friendship.

❧

Thank you to all the battalions of Healers
who have joined forces with us.

❧

Thank you first and last to the
Children of the Future.

Love, Life and Light,

William

FOREWORD

My life changed dramatically, drastically, and irrevocably on November 17, 2005. That was my death day and re-birthday. The external event was surgical removal of a glioblastoma multiforme tumor phase IV from the left occipital-parietal lobe of my cranium. Though I was unconscious during surgery, what I experienced was transcendent, like being turned inside out and hovering in timelessness, between this world and the life after life, and returning to here and now—changed forever. What sounds like a cliché describes literally what I felt.

Before I begin to describe my spiritual quest in the six directions with cancer as my adversary/companion, it would be wise to establish home base: Hawthorne Valley. I call it "Happy Valley." The vital spirit of this place, *genius loci*, is a key player in the story that follows, providing an ever-changing tapestry of seasons, flora, fauna, streams, rocks, trees, children, characters, festivals and community that are the enduring life of the valley.

Life-threatening illness greatly intensifies love of life. For the past three decades, I have been extraordinarily blessed to count myself among the pioneer teachers and farmers cooperating to build up, by the sweat of our brows, a unique and lively school on a biodynamic dairy farm—Hawthorne Valley Farm. We are located in the historic Hudson River Valley in Columbia County, upstate New York, 150 miles due north of New York City and fifteen miles east of the old whaling town of Hudson and the Hudson River.

The farm is nestled between forested ridges of bedrock shale in the foothills of the Taconic Range, just west of the more famous Berkshires that form the border between New York State and Massachusetts to the east. The rock ridges are blue in winter, tones of green in spring and summer, and ablaze with fiery color in fall. The hills are covered with maples, oaks, hickories, poplars, hemlocks, white pines, and birches. Animals of all kinds have reclaimed the overgrown forest—squirrels, chipmunks, raccoons, martens, foxes, coyotes, beaver, a few bear, and too many deer to count. A great variety of birds also find this place to their liking: owls, eagles, crows, martins, robins, thrushes, goldfinches, red-winged blackbirds, chickadees, grackles, sparrows, redbirds, blue-birds, orioles, tufted titmice, wrens, vultures, blue jays, herons, grouse, and turkeys. Let's not overlook smiling tree frogs, newts, salamanders, toads, tadpoles, and grumpy snapping turtles. We won't delve into the vast inventory of insects and colorful butter-flies or pesky flies, but we must give thanks for the golden bless-ings of the honeybee, without which…nothing.

A herd of fifty-plus brown Swiss dairy cows enjoys cropping the grass. The ruminating "ladies" are our pride and joy, offering raw milk, which is sold through the Farm Store in "downtown" Harlemville, as well as creamy yogurt, and several kinds of cheese. Ten acres of market garden cover the bottomland. The biodynami-cally grown produce is seasonally available at the Farm Store. The farm also supplies top quality food to a Community Supported Agriculture (CSA) network of shareholders. Delicious, wholesome breads are freshly baked daily in our own bakery; aged cheese, creamy yogurt, and fresh produce are trucked down to the Union Square Market in New York City twice each week. No pesticides or herbicides have touched our fields for thirty-five years. Farmer's gold, composted manure enriching the fields, is our endowment fund. Aging wheels of cheese in the vault constitute our Swiss bank account. We have been pioneers in biodynamic agriculture in our region and were among the founding members of the Columbia Land Conservancy.

Next to the farm, based in the old farmhouse, is the Visit-ing Students Program of environmental education. From humble beginnings, now more than five hundred students each year from twenty-six schools, come for a week at a time to work on the farm, gather eggs, haul manure, pick up rocks, plant seeds, curry cows, feed slops and whey to the pigs, explore the woods, weed gardens, bake bread, prepare and serve meals, and connect with Mother Earth. Most students consider the farm trip the highlight of their educational career!

Across the street from the farmhouse is Hawthorne Valley School. It now has an enrollment of more than three hundred students, kindergarten through twelfth grade. When I came as a new class teacher in 1976, there were sixty-five children K-6. Eleven were in my first class of first graders. The school started off in a house that had belonged to a minister, and it was purchased after his death for $7,000. In a way, I was a "natural" as a teacher, because I was interested in everything. But "ninety percent of success in life is just showing up." In the great scheme of things, all education is self-education. We are all students of life, for life.

To make sense of this story, as well as the pivotal role of the *Children of the Future,* a few more words of context will be helpful before taking the plunge. Hawthorne Valley School is a Waldorf, or Rudolf Steiner, school. All Waldorf schools, about seven hundred worldwide, are inspired by the educational insights of Rudolf Steiner. From his spiritual scientific research, Steiner stimulated cultural renewal in a number of fields, including education (general and special), agriculture, medicine, economics, architecture, science, philosophy, religion, and the arts. The schools are diverse, adapting themselves to many different cultures across the globe. They are independent and autonomous, but share a common philosophy. Essential features of the philosophy include:

- A keen interest in and study of each child in the teacher's care;
- An on-going study of human development, especially as it relates to a teacher's specific classes;
- A commitment to community building and positive collegial working;
- A wide interest in a teacher's subject area and in the world as a whole;
- A commitment by the teacher to the cultivation of her/his own creative sources;
- An active practice of self-reflection by the teacher.

In the 1960s, a small group of pioneer educators, farmers, and artists who had been connected with building up the Rudolf Steiner School in New York City (founded in 1929) envisioned the kind of place Hawthorne Valley has since become. They foresaw a social organism in a natural environment that combined education, agriculture, and the arts. The founding impulse is epitomized in the words of Karl Ege taken from *An Evident Need of Our Time:*

> What we are founding here is a seed—the seed of a living organism. This organism is essentially threefold—pedagogical, artistic and agricultural—as reflections of thought, feeling and will. Each needs the others if the whole is to flourish. All are interrelated. But just as the life of the functioning body is more than the sum of its parts, so the evolving life of the whole Farm School *community* constitutes, in reality, a greater entity—the expression of its spiritual task.
>
> It is this task that is community building. It is out of a common cultural and social striving in pursuit of this spiritual goal, which is in the widest sense educational, that a humanly worthy and satisfying work together as a larger expanding community will be wrought. For young and old alike, this work together will create a place in which to *become*, in the true sense, a full human being.

For my wife Andy and me, a young couple setting out in life in 1976, Hawthorne Valley provided an ideal setting in which to raise our family and provide Waldorf education for our daughters. Unfortunately, no one had heard of Waldorf education, biodynamic agriculture, or Rudolf Steiner in our neck of the woods—or anywhere else for that matter. Unencumbered by prior experience, with a twelve-month crash course in Waldorf education under my belt, I joined a few colleagues who were carving a school out of the wilderness. Learn by doing is a fundamental Waldorf principle, so that is what we did. It turns out that the work of building up a school never lets up. The *ideals* build the school; we just supply the helping hands.

A cooperative, "can-do" power of initiative impelled us forward. The soil was rocky, the site remote, the money scarce, and the neighboring communities skeptical, but the will to work was strong and the ideal a brilliant guiding star. The motive power to do what needed to be done came from the children. Many parents share the feeling of being led to Waldorf education by their children. Somehow, children have the mysterious ability to organize life around their future needs and aspirations.

Until the responsibilities of family life gradually dawned on me, I had been a back-to-the-land hippie and aspiring wood carver in New Mexico. After my teacher training, I was transformed into an earnest but innocent novice on the school side of the road. Enthusiasm and midnight oil had to take the place of insight or experience. I was a better carpenter than teacher, but not a great carpenter either. I was trying to compensate for gaping holes in my own education, like: What is the role of the Will? The children had to teach me everything. The hard way. The parents had a hand in it, too! But I was cheerful, patient, and willing to learn. And I enjoyed, appreciated, and recognized the children for who they were. I worked harmoniously and cooperatively with parents and colleagues united in common striving. Somehow I managed to keep my balance and enthusiasm through many years of apprenticeship. My strong suit was writing plays and telling stories. I was most interested in people of all kinds and characters.

When our younger daughter Rosie was old enough for kindergarten, Andy joined the faculty as assistant to kindergarten teacher Astrid Barnes. Within two years, she had her own kindergarten and has been teaching ever since—about twenty-six years in all. Waldorf kindergartens, with their festivals and puppets, deserve their own book.*

I was a Waldorf "Class Teacher," which is more a calling than a profession. As class teacher, a group of children was entrusted to my care for eight years. Now, there is a leap of faith! We grew with the transformations of the curriculum, from the fairy tales

---

* See, for example, *What Is a Waldorf Kindergarten?* (SteinerBooks, 2007), compiled and introduced by Sharifa Oppenheimer and edited by Joan Almon, both longtime Waldorf kindergarten teachers.

and form drawings in the first grade, through science, math, and history in the eighth grade. There is no repetition of material from the previous year by compartmentalized specialists; the Waldorf method is a continuously evolving, creative process. This means that the teacher is constantly assimilating and forming the material that is presented orally to the students. This then becomes the primary material of the students' work and practice. They are not presented with textbooks, homework sheets, tests, or freeze-dried lessons. Instead, they create their own main lesson books based on the subjects surveyed through engaged dialogue. It is a living education. I repeated this eight-year cycle four times.

The class teacher collaborates with other colleagues, who teach special subjects such as French, German, handwork, eurythmy (an art of movement), music, physical education, gardening projects, and form drawing. A central goal of this form of education is to involve the students and their teachers fully in a creative process that integrates thinking, feeling, and willing. The gradual awakening and balancing of these soul capacities of head, heart, and hand lead to discovering, releasing, and realizing our full human potential. The depth, breadth, and wisdom of the cumulative curriculum instill lifelong love of learning, love of beauty, reverence for the earth, practical skill, power of initiative, and compassion for our fellow human beings. These moral qualities are the common possession of all peoples and all children. Through them we find ourselves in the world and the world in our Self.

Let that serve as background for the story about to begin.

In the air I hear an overarching melody of grace: "I once was lost, but now I'm found...." I am both terminally ill and vitally alive. This book is offered to all who have undergone or been touched by serious illness of any kind, not just cancer; and who seek to find their individual path through that dark forest back into the shining light of day.

A close friend who died of cancer not long ago was cooking breakfast at the stove. She stopped what she was doing and turned pointedly to me (in recovery and in suspense about my cancer's resurgence) and said, "Aside from marrying my husband, John, cancer is the best thing that ever happened to me." I knew exactly what she meant. We laughed. Perhaps only a cancer patient can know the import of those words. They do not mean that she did not suffer. Her suffering was heart-wrenching. She was young, about forty, beautiful, vivacious, feisty, determined to overcome the wasting away caused by illness. Nonetheless, she affirmed "I have learned so much!" Her gratitude toward life was radiant. Life!

Cancer is an illness that has touched millions of people one way or another. Each person touched becomes a seeker. Cancer is not just the Grim Reaper, stalking through the land with his scythe. Cancer is a mirror holding up a picture of our time. It carries vital life and death messages for us that we urgently wish to decipher. The most powerful of these is the healing power of love. The gentle influence of love does not necessarily stop or indefinitely delay the spread of cancer, though that is also a miraculous possibility and potent hope. But love is the great healer of body, soul, and spirit, both in life and in life after death. Without the abundant love I have received, I would not be able to give back this story. Now the journey begins.

TRAVELING LIGHT

OWL SACRIFICE

SISTER OWL, WISE SPIRIT messenger, night guardian—guide my way through the shadows of death to newborn life.

"Whooo, whooo wanders at midnight?"
"I."
"Why?"
"To find my way."
"Tooo?
"To who I am"
"I will guide you."
"Is it far?
"Over the mountains, over the sea,
Over the moon, to the rising sun."

Perfect! Heading toward Grand Menan, New Brunswick, skirting the inlets of the Bay of Fundy. Rolling through hemlock and spruce woods. Sea air. School's out, summer teaching's over. Freedom, free time. Time to breathe in the sea air, time to walk the cliffs and coves, time to write, read, eat, nap. Time to *be*. Northern clarity. Perfect!

In all that forested wilderness, in all that ocean of air, at an ordained moment, the gray owl, intent, swoops silently. There is no avoiding this rendezvous. *Wake!* ***Impact!*** *Death!*

I had killed the owl. It was a bolt from the blue, unavoidable, suicidal. There was no one else on the road. Andy and I were thunderstruck, shaken. I, who brake for frogs, had inadvertently snuffed out in an instant a creature so magnificent and mysterious. In broad daylight. Why? Replay. Gliding in from the periphery, the owl swooped low from the left, directly into our path. Blindsided.

There was no turning around — no respectful woodland burial, no incense offering, only self-recrimination and futile wishing it had not happened. Random? I don't think so. Omen of what? We were profoundly disturbed by this accident. Owl: totem of wisdom, wakefulness, mystery, magic, single-minded attention.

This incident from the summer of 2005 could easily have been repressed if it had not become the herald of this story.

Four months after striking the owl, on November 10, shortly after Halloween, I was diagnosed with brain cancer. *Glioblastoma multiforme.* Immediate surgery mandatory. Within a month we would discover that this cancer was aggressive and malignant. A killer.

Flashback: When I started as a Waldorf teacher with my first first grade in 1976, my repertoire of poems and stories was pitifully small. Dealing with the energy of eleven seven-year olds in a tiny room in a pioneering school gave me a headache every day. My life forces were drained before I knew what to call them. Daily naps were crucial to survival. Rudolf Copple was the wise, seventy-two-year-old mentor of our school at the time. He taught me this nursery rhyme that proved useful to calm an excited class:

> A wise old owl sat in an oak.
> The more he heard, the less he spoke.
> The less he spoke, the more he heard.
> Let's all be like that wise old bird.

Now I have entered the owl's realm. My listening is all-encompassing. My eyes are wide. I am airborne.

My life changed in the instant we learned of my brain cancer. I had been a Waldorf class teacher at Hawthorne Valley School for thirty years. That career, to which I had dedicated my adult life, came to an abrupt close on November 17, 2005, the day of my surgery. Now what was I? Who was I, stripped of my professional identity? I was bearer of a particularly virulent brain cancer en route to Albany Medical Center. I was no longer a teacher. I was a student. Cancer was now my nemesis and, as I discovered, my teacher. I had much to learn.

HALLOWEEN

I REMEMBER VIVIDLY THAT, TWENTY-EIGHT years ago, our first daughter Claire and I—owl and wizard—wandered through the neighborhood when she was in first grade one Halloween. Her costume was simple, a blanket pinned to make wings over her arms and a horned owl mask with wise eyes, like hers, that I made for her from a brown paper bag. Oh, the cuteness and simplicity of old timey ways. Ooooo, the mystery of the cold, starry night.

Thirty years later, wizard again, what am I doing up in a tree at my age (then fifty-nine) in the dark? I am wearing a black robe, sporting a lengthy beard, and wearing a wizard's broad brimmed hat. Skeletons, vampires, pirates, princesses, gypsies, hoboes, gangsters, witches, owls, black cats, bats, lions, fairies, and devils have been loosed into the dark forest. All Hallows' Eve, preceding All Souls' Day and All Saints' Day, the veil between this world and the spiritual world is threadbare. This is when the spirits of the dead come close to their remembered earthly home. Bare trees hold up bony fingers to the moon. The dried corpses of the leaves rattle. Flaming colors of a week before are now ash. The "dark is rising." The northern hemisphere is descending into winter's starry night. The untamed nature spirits, demons, tricksters, trolls, hobgoblins, and formless fears must be cleansed away for the light to be reborn.

We take Halloween seriously in Hawthorne Valley. There are jack-o'-lanterns illuminating the path across the bridge to the wizard riddle master, who wonders what on earth he is doing. Maybe Baba Yaga, the story-telling witch who appears every year at this time, could help, but she has customers already in the glowing candlelight and is too far away. Little do I realize that the beast is within, gnawing on the roots of the World Tree, and growing unchecked. This is ten days before I will be diagnosed. At some submerged level of consciousness, I must be aware that the deadly creature is growing. Like Gandalf in Moria, the wizard will soon be in a fight for his life against the baleful Balrog. Gandalf's command reverberates in the abyss, **"You shall not pass!"**

But at this point the wizard, who grudgingly came to the festival when he wanted to stay at home, is warming to his task. Little denizens of the night, flanked by torches, gaze upward at the lantern-lit wise man. They are the seekers on a night journey full of surprises. I pretend I have all the answers, but soon I will have no answers, only unanswerable, haunting questions. The Great Riddle Master in the sky may or may not answer my questions. Perhaps I don't even know what questions to ask. Certainly some dark questions I don't want answered. But my immediate task was clear. I would do the asking, and the wee creatures of the night would guess the answer, if they were up to the challenge and wanted a treat from the wizard.

> *In a marble hall white as milk*
> *Lined with skin as soft as silk*
> *Within a fountain crystal-clear*
> *A golden apple doth appear.*
> *No doors there are to this stronghold,*
> *Yet thieves break in to steal its gold.*

> *No sooner spoken than broken.*

> *The greater it is*
> *The less you see of it.*

> *At night they come without being fetched,*
> *And by day they are lost without being stolen.*

> *A very pretty thing am I,*
> *Fluttering in the pale-blue sky.*
> *Delicate, fragile on the wing,*
> *Indeed I am a pretty thing.*

> *What is it that makes tears without sorrow*
> *and takes its journey to heaven?*

Silence, an egg, darkness, stars, butterfly, smoke—all these "kennings" come from the realm where meaning is found, where riddles light up, where one thing dissolves into another. You can seek the meaning if you keep to the mean, and are never mean, if you know what I mean. The supplicant must find the key of the kingdom of imagination before the door to knowledge opens.

"The greater it is, the less you see of it." Darkness. Nowhere are we more in the dark than before the greatest riddles: life and death. Now with illness as my guide I have entered a realm reverberating with revelations. The nut of habit cracks open. I have become the seed which must die to be reborn. Brother Death becomes the great teacher for the meaning of life. Even these children's riddles and nursery rhymes become important, filled with import. *"Ring around the rosey, a pocket full of posies, ashes, ashes, we all fall down."* Owl guardian, give me wise new eyes for butterflies. I know that they, enduring the chaos of metamorphosis, emerge like Lazarus from the tomb, transformed from caterpillar to creature of the light and air. They are a true picture of the death and resurrection of the soul. This is why psyche means both soul and butterfly. May I, on the edge between this world and the beyond belatedly learn to read directly from the Book of Life the song of creation. The script, "the Logos structure of the universe," is an open secret. Musing, listening to the muse, music, being amused, are portals through the looking glass of mere perception, mirror reflection into living dialogue with nature. *Natura* speaks. Each pebble has a story to tell to those with ears to hear and eyes to see. "To one who is silent, even the mute stones speak." The word "poetry" springs from the babbling of a brook. The rustling of the wind through the trees of the sacred grove whispers inklings and bodings. The incantations of poetry and puzzling riddles awaken us. Metaphor, the magical transformation from seeming to being, frees us from our "literal" ("on the shore") mindedness. Now is the time to set sail on the ocean of meanings. The "wind" (*pneuma, ruach, spiritus*) fills our sails with the breath of inspiration. Imagination holds the rudder through storm and calm on this sea as guiding constellations, beings and powers wheel across the midnight sky.

I enjoyed being up the tree. It was an improv situation: anything can happen. Just like life. The format is simple. Ask a question, find the answer, receive a reward. No answer, no ginger candy (more burning than sweet). At the time, my only question was "What am I doing up this tree?" In a few more days branching questions proliferated like the cancer itself, around the vortex center, the existential question: would I live or die? The answer is: both. When? No telling. The jury is still out.

MAGNETIC RESONATING IMAGERY

THE SECOND WEEK OF November I had a persistent head and neck ache. I asked my teaching intern in my fourth grade class to keep an eye on me, I wasn't feeling quite myself. My thoughts were trailing off, I wrote the same phrase on the board twice, I needed to sit down. I thought I was having a relapse of a flu from three weeks before. Andy had noticed I was more absent-minded (than usual). She did not like these headaches, rare for me, and my energy was down. It was worrisome that I had difficulty typing out a set of arithmetic problems. Searching for keys, we speculated maybe I had Lyme disease. After school on Monday, late afternoon, I drove to my friend Dr. Steve Kaufman for a blood test and a check up. He said, "It could be Lyme disease or the flu again, but let's eliminate other possibilities." Dr. Kaufman's twenty-five years of emergency room service made him cautious. "Go get an MRI in Hudson." His intervention at this moment likely saved my life. (For how long only the Riddle Master knows.)

Andy had known for days that something was up. A week before, as I laid a treasure hunt out for the fourth graders before school, I had snapped at her, "Don't talk to me now, I'm trying to get these clues laid out." I was confused and disoriented. Should clue number nine go under the bridge in the eighth spot to lead on…or does clue eight go in the eighth spot and nine in the ninth? I couldn't decipher my own treasure map pinpointing the locations. Uncharacteristically, I was brusque again a week later: " Look, I'm trying to take care of all these errands as fast as I can. Yes, I'm going to the doctor. Yes, I can drive myself. I just have a lot of things on my plate." (or THING on my mind).

So, following Dr. Kaufman's advice, I drove to Hudson, Wednesday on a late afternoon through a deluge. Stripped of all metal, gowned, I padded across the tile floor in hospital issue non-slip socklets. I entered the million dollar marvel of the Magnetic-Resonance-Imaging (MRI) machine. Foam blocks were pushed against my ears (not tightly enough as it turned out). Head immobilizer down. Check. Periscope up. Check. I glided into my metallic coffin. Technician to sound booth, tin can intercom on. Check. Trusting William prays to the benevolent powers that he be found free and clear….

Blast off! A VERY LOUD SOUND instantaneously juiced my adrenals into overdrive: fight, flight, or freeze. Freeze seemed to be the best and only option.

KLANG…CLICK…CLICK…CLICK…CLICK….CLICK…
KLANG…CLICK…CLICK…CLICK…CLICK….CLICK…
KLANG…CLICK…CLICK…CLICK…CLICK….CLICK…

Relax! Yeh, I'm OK with this. I'm not claustrophobic. Not me. I'm in the Lord's hands. God, that's loud! There are better ear plugs for a buck at the hardware store than these foam blocks…. I think the technician left too much air space…. Where is the volume control?…. Relax…. Who thought up this gadget?…. GE…. product placement…. Progress is our most important product…. Ronald Reagan…. Raygun…. Strategic Defense Initiative…. Trust in the guidance of spiritual beings….The KLANG of the anvil chorus…." Swart smirched smiths drive me to death with the din of their dents"…. ***KLANG!***

(*Disembodied voice through tin can intercom from the control/sound booth: "You all right in there?"*)

"No problemo. It's just a little loud. Is there a volume control anywhere? *Am I bleeding from my ear drums?... Does anyone ever freak out in here?... Bring it on. Dear Lord, I entrust myself to your care.*

GRUNK...DUT...DUT...DUT...DUT...DUT...DUT
GRUNK...DUT...DUT...DUT...DUT...DUT...DUT
GRUNK...DUT...DUT...DUT...DUT...DUT...DUT

It's the same old song with a different meaning since you been gone.... Have mercy on me.... Thy light let it enlighten the sphere of my thinking...maybe they're just piping in this sound and charging a couple grand.... I wonder what my health insurance policy says about MRIs...what do forty-five million people do without health insurance? Hope for the best?.... Relax.... Why do they keep it so cold in here?

Tin can intercom, "How're we doing in there, Mr. Ward?"

What do you mean "we," Kemosabe? Fine (*always compliant*). *All systems go. Ready for liftoff....* "Fear, the mind destroyer"...."I pray the Lord my soul to keep".... *I'm going to be all right.... Maybe I should stay home tomorrow and kick this flu...hate to miss a day....* "When in the morning light I wake, help me the path of Love to take...."

A few more Ozifying-mechano-magneto roundelays from the gizmo and the human subject emerges into the fluorescent light of night. "There you are, that's all there is to it. Stop by for the images in the morning."

I had much to ponder on the ride home. Let's see now, which way is home? I drove on auto pilot, took an aspirin, and fell asleep. I doubt Andy did.

SAINT MARTIN'S DAY

THE NEXT DAY, "COINCIDENTALLY" (a premise that I give little credence to), November 11, Veterans Day, is also the Day of the Dead. Traditionally we have a pageant at Hawthorne Valley where first to third graders perform the story of the compassionate soldier Martin who cuts his cloak in two to share with a homeless wanderer. This saves the beggar's life. Martin sleeps that night on the ground. He has a heavenly vision that reveals he had shared his cloak with the Son of Man who now gives Martin a cloak of light:

CHORUS OF ANGELS, BEGGARS, AND THE SON OF MAN:

> Martin, you so loved me, your blood red robe you gave.
> By your brotherly kindness this beggar's life you saved.
> Now and for all time to come, your cloak is woven whole
> Of what can never tear nor fade and never will grow old.
> Because you gave your cloak away, it ever will increase.
> Of courage it is made, and life and love and peace.

Third graders portray the soldiers who, except for Martin, ignore the beggar. Second graders are the cold beggars with one among them as Everyman in need. The first graders are angels who descend from heavenly heights and raise Martin up to meet the Son of Man face to face.

The pageant, which I had written perhaps fifteen years ago, is performed annually at this melancholy time of year. I had never missed it, but I would not see it this year. I was in Albany Medical Center. Soon I would receive a robe of light.

Andy left her Parent-Child class immediately when she got the call from Dr. Kaufman on Thursday morning. "Get him to Albany for further tests." The parents were abruptly left in charge. "What's up with William?" swept through the school. I had taken a sick day (a great rarity in my many years of teaching) and had slept in. Andy drove me to Albany Medical Center for a battery of tests: blood test, MRI with injected contrast, and a full body CT scan. After a busy morning we would review the images with a specialist. Andy and I held hands. Mine were cold, hers were warm. Minds racing. Keep the faith. *Breathe.*

After the MRIs and CT scan, we waited for a review. I was given Dilantin to prevent the possibility of epileptic seizure resulting from the rapid swelling of the brain before and after surgery. Under the influence, I could hardly follow what the neurologist was saying. The gist was that the MRI images showed a plum-sized tumor on the left parietal-occipital region of my brain. Once it was surgically removed the tissue would be analyzed to determine whether it was *malignant* or *benign*. "Malignant: 1a; *obsolete*: MALCONTENT, DISAFFECTED; b: evil in nature, influence, or effect: INJURIOUS; c: passionately and relentlessly malevolent: aggressively malicious; 2: tending to produce death or deterioration: tending to infiltrate, metastasize, and terminate, fatally <malignant tumor>.... Benign *from bene+gigni*, well-born; 1: of a gentle disposition: GRACIOUS < a benign teacher [!]> 2a: showing kindness and gentleness; b: FAVORABLE; 3: of a mild character < a benign tumor >" (*Webster's New Collegiate Dictionary*).

Just because I'm paranoid doesn't mean something isn't trying to kill me. In this case it is an uninvited guest in the cauliflower of my brain, proliferating exponentially with no consideration for its host, me.

"But even uninvited guests bring gifts," a survivor told me later. Actually, I was not paranoid. Rather than feeling under siege from within, I felt substantially protected. In my rapidly evolving understanding of and speculation about my humble but intense place in the universe, I sensed I was being guided. My unfolding life was being witnessed, powerfully but with surprising detachment by myself. And not only by me from the inside, but witnessed by dear Andy as closest empathetic participant, my daughters and their partners, and by my compassionate community. Most inwardly, my true Self, from whom no thought is hidden, held the panorama of my life in reverence.

Admittedly, this could be a problem for those of us intent upon concealing certain things, even from our selves. Cancer to the rescue. Nothing can be concealed any longer. Viscera and tissue will be on display. My guardian, however, beholds me as I am with the eyes of mercy, love, forgiveness, blessing, and healing. This gentle brother loves me more than I love myself. In true confession mode, despite my façade of confidence, I would have to admit that I do not love myself. I am too aware of my weaknesses and shadow. No, I long for the unconditional love of a mother for her vulnerable child but feel ever unworthy. Welcome to the human condition.

At this point in the story I am still holding Andy's hand, trying to understand what the radiologist is saying, as we face my brain surgery, the possibility of the cancer being fatal, or the possibility of permanent impairment of my movement and speech centers. Speech center! Wait a minute. I need that. Too ironic. Who is writing the script? Either do me in or make me a survivor, but please don't take away the power of speech. Bargaining with unseen powers, I vow never to take speech for granted again. The peace of silence had not yet dawned in me.

Meanwhile, during the "debriefing" (talk about a phrase rife with humorous implications) something very interesting is occupying my attention. The succession of MRI cross sections displayed on the "terminal" (pardon the expression) are to me unmistakably demonic. Through the wizardry of the MRI technique, layers of my brain, usually discretely hidden in the Platonic cave of the skull, are revealed as ghostly, if not ghastly, images. There is the tumor showing white because of the "contrast" injection that distinguishes it from the gray matter and negative (in every sense of the word) quality of the images. Bizarrely beautiful, each symmetrical cross-section has the physiognomy of a bat or demon. It's amusing in a macabre way, fascinating, like a Rorschach test, metamorphosing through the levels but staying with the same gargoyle vibe. This is, after all, the Day of the Dead in the Place of the Skull.

Long-Lost Friend

I was to remain in the hospital for observation. We were informed that inflammation, headaches, the swelling pressure of edema in the brain cavity, and potential seizures were possible consequences of the growing tumor.

The Writer of the Script still being written had already subliminally prophesied to me that the tumor was malignant. A figment of my Dilantin-suffused imagination promoted this dangerous possibility: "Go with the more dramatic story. Forget 'Tumor Benign!' No punch. 'Ward Recovers and Resumes Teaching Career,' so what, who cares? 'Ward Dies But Lives!' This has market appeal. The bobble head spin-off alone, plus pharmaceutical endorsements will set you up for life...as short as that may be."

I command, *Begone, Figment, Ferret Voice of Doom!*

Can the patient, referring to myself from the safer vantage point of the third person, quickly grow wings and cross unscathed to the further shore? Doubtful, too easy, escapist fantasy, irresponsible cop out. No. This is real life. *It is initiation time.* I felt I would now go through something dark and light and deep and high.

Andy kept vigil in my hospital room all night. That must have been one looong night. She had to be brave and do the worrying for two, since I, knocked out, was neglecting my share. When I woke, I puked my guts out as a reaction to the Dilantin (ominous name). No seizure though. That reminds me of a joke: "What are you doing with that fly whisk?" "Keeping elephants away." "How do you know it works." "You see any elephants?" From my reaction we concluded that the Dilantin was too strong for a clean liver like myself, used to nothing stronger than Italian roast coffee and a tad of dark organic chocolate (for the anti-oxidants, whatever they are). They switched me to brand B.

Andy spent Friday waiting, watching me sleep it off and expecting momentarily for the neurosurgeon to give us an update of what to expect and when. No one came. They were in surgery all day. Finally they appeared, like *Right Stuff* demigods in the hierarchy of high-tech medicine: Dr. German (I already felt better) and Dr. Friedlich ("Dr. Peaceful"). If you're going to have brain surgery go with a germ-free German every time. The training, the posture, the knowledge, the precision, the sense of order, the objectivity. Think Mercedes, BMW, Bosch. No fun-loving, volatile Italian barbers redolent with olive oil, chianti, and garlic need apply. Step aside made-in-China surgical instruments, give me Solingen. Place with confidence the surgical steel of the cranial circular saw in the hands of a skilled German craftsman. Certainly the angels were watching over me with a team like this. We had six more days till zero hour.

Andy was encouraged to go home, take a shower, and get some rest and a change of clothes. I would remain under observation. While home she also called our doctor, Margaretha Hertle, who would now be supervising my post-surgical treatment. Andy informed Margaretha the surgery would be in a week, November 17. Our friend Branko Furst, a highly respected anesthesiologist at Albany Medical Center, was already confirming that we had the best possible team. He came to visit me and assured us he would greet us at the door at dawn the day of surgery and accompany us through prep. After surgery the tumor tissue would be analyzed for malignancy. Until then, given my reaction to the Dilantin, it was advised that I be kept under observation in the neuro ward (or should I say "neuro Ward").

When Andy told Dr. Hertle that they wanted to keep me in the neuro ward, she said, "Get him out of there! You can't get well in a hospital. He needs rest at home in his own bed before surgery." Margaretha, also of German ancestry, is decisive. That's why we like her.

Before Andy returned from home to the hospital the following day, she made one phone call in particular. (The deluge of messages from the four quarters was just beginning.) My childhood best friend, Tom Mollison, "just happened to be passing through." His grandson Jeremy left a message on our phone and a number where they could be reached. Could they swing by for a visit? They were on an expedition to the Baseball Hall of Fame in Cooperstown. Andy called back, "William's in Albany Medical Center. He'll have brain surgery on Thursday. He'll be so glad to see you, Tom. Will he be surprised!"

"This was no dream; I lay broad waking..." (Master Fulke Grevell). I was astounded to see my dear, wise friend Tom in my hospital room in Albany. His presence was too impossibly significant to be mere coincidence. The divine Author was beginning to call in the cast for the last farewell, or rallying the forces of karmic brotherhood for a last minute save.

Until the summer before, I had not seen Tom since my mother's funeral in 1994. Living near her, he had been a stand-in for me as surrogate son and was the last person my mother spoke with before inviting him to leave so she could lie down...and die peacefully at home.

Even with this strong connection, Tom and I had lost touch. When the Association of Waldorf Schools of North America had its teachers' conference in Ann Arbor, Michigan, in August of 2005, three months before the detection of my illness, on a whim or guided premonition, I saw an opportunity to visit my childhood home, pay my respects at my parents' grave, and visit Tom. At that time the notion of my own demise was preposterous. But I was being stalked already. I had learned Tom had Parkinson's disease. He was in his fifth year. The day I arrived in Niles, Michigan, was the day he had given up his practice as a CPA after about thirty-five years. We reminisced about many things from our childhood.

We were the Dagger Doubles, a secret club with two members.

Our exploits included riding bicycles at top speed down hill, getting in shape, holding marble races, playing marathon board games for days with huge sums of money, swinging on vines in Mickey's woods, playing poker, playing cops and robbers, sleeping over, playing cowboys and Indians, emerging victorious from big time wrestling with the Union Street Lilliputians, camping out in the playhouse, shooting baskets, playing chess, collecting chestnuts, trading baseball cards, playing kick the can, practicing for Little League, looking for bugs, going on expeditions beyond the tracks, building forts of snow, leaves, and sticks, and holding our breath under water till we were ready to burst. Completing this cycle of activities, we would begin again. We were inseparable. Tom blames me for his lifelong love of golf, something I gave up at age twelve with a sore back and an incurable slice.

Now we were in the same room fifty years later, Tom with Parkinson's, me preparing for brain surgery. When I had visited Niles in the summer, Tom had said with a depth and equanimity that put me in awe: "I'm grateful for my illness. I have become a teacher through being dependent on the support of others. I have learned a great deal about the power of love and prayer. I'm in a partnership with people, I receive and others give. Some people don't get it, but most do." Tom, my friend, had come to see me. Dear Author who continues to write *William Ward: This Is Your Life!* Thank you for letting me grow up with my friend Tom, thank you for bringing him here, now.

These words of Novalis echo those of my wise friend, Tom:

> The heart is the key to life and the world. If our life
>   is as precarious
> as it is, it is so only in order that we should love and
>   need one
> another. Because of the fact that we are each of us
>   insufficient, we
> become open to the intervention of another, and it is
>   this intervention
> which is the goal. When we are ill, others must look
>   after us; and only
> they can do so. From this point of view, Christ is
>   indisputably the key
> to the world.

PRELUDE

Big brother Dave with his partner Barbara, alerted by Andy, rolled into the hospital Saturday afternoon from Rector, Pennsylvania. With Dave at my right hand, as he always has been before, surely all would be well. And Barbara's relentless positivity and empathy were a great support for Andy and me as we were trying to find the Ground beneath our feet. Brother Dave inspires confidence. He's a college professor, antique race car restorer and enthusiast, Joyce scholar, playwright, historian, and film authority. He and I are the sole survivors of a dead-end branch of the ancient Ward lineage (but that's another story). Here is a Mensch to have in your corner.

MEANWHILE, I FANTASIZE WILEY COYOTE monomaniacally intent on catching the Road Runner. Wiley goes over the canyon's edge into thin air in hot pursuit. Hovering cloud high, he looks down and realizes nothing is holding him up. The shock of this recognition precipitates his fall. He claws the air as he descends into the vanishing point of the abyss. A small puff of dust announces his return to terra firma. Flattened into two dimensions, he rises from the dust and continues his eternal pursuit of his nemesis.

Similarly, I'm in thin air, looking down, having just realized this is no dream. My nemesis is pursuing me. My name is William. I have a potentially fatal brain tumor. The karmic brotherhood-sisterhood of fellow wayfarers are beginning to form around this body, this soul, this spirit at the moment of trial.

Word had spread far and wide around the school community that I would have surgery Thursday. My class was substituted by two long-time friends—kind-hearted Stuart Summer, the eighth grade teacher, and my dear friend Candace Christiansen, who taught high school chemistry and weaving at our school.

Stuart could substitute because someone was teaching his class the current block. He made cards with the class for me, putting on the board his own drawing that showed a good likeness of me with a huge smiling angel hovering behind me placing both hands upon my head. The message from this image beaming at me from the living room wall was "All is well, you are in good hands." When it was clear I would be out for a while, Candace Christiansen jumped in. Her granddaughter Kaulini was in the class. She was a grandmother to all the children and a good woman to have in your corner in a health crisis. She'd been through it all. She was first to visit us in the hospital with her husband Thomas Locker. We had visited Thomas a couple years before when he went under the knife for quadruple by-pass heart surgery. He had nearly died en route to the hospital and told me later of his near-death experience. His paintings of the spirit in nature had always been an inspiration to all those who know and love his children's books. I couldn't grasp his vision then, but his paintings, always breathtakingly beautiful, had crossed into the sublime. Candace is as down-to-earth practical as Thomas is a philosopher-artist. In addition to teaching, she throws pots and collaborates with Thomas.

My hospital visit to them two years ago was now mirrored by their support for me in my need. "One good turn deserves another," the fairy tale says. Now, dear friends were by my side. Thomas, who has an artist's soul and sensitivity, could barely speak knowing exactly what I must be going through. Candace with her photographic memory, medical knowledge, and intimate familiarity with hospitals was radiating confidence in the outcome, whatever she may have been thinking inwardly. "They found the tumor early, it's accessible to surgery, they'll cut it out, you'll be home before you know it. Standard operating procedure. These guys are amazing. Everybody is praying for you. Let us know. Whatever you need, we'll do. Call." But Thomas's soulful eyes were filled with tears.

Medicine Wheel

The clan gathered. To me, our daughters in family mythology are like Snow White and Rose Red. Claire, the elder, is contemplative, imaginative, artistic, melancholic. Rosie, the younger, is energetic, decisive, straightforward, and courageously honest with herself and others. They are as different as can be, complementary and supportive of each other through thick and thin. Claire's husband Josh is a gifted guitarist and songwriter, wired with the nervous energy of the Big City, hilariously funny, with great people skills. Rose's partner Billy is a man of will and action, hardworking, athletic, and upright. His smile is like sunshine. Then there is OTTO. This is our grandson. He is a Child of the Future, but what that really means, I will soon KNOW.

We held council with one another. Our love and appreciation for each other grew wider and deeper knowing that a sword, or rather a buzz saw, hung over my head. It seemed as if, behind our masks, I could see the soul struggles of each of us confronting the uncertainties of my surgery and the indefinite future. In the limbo of waiting, we were transparent to each other. We were in a lifeboat, trying to be brave, hoping for rescue, riding on swells and troughs of anxiety, fear, hope, devotion, laughter, courage, faith, acceptance, anger, denial, openness, confidence. Choppy seas. But there was also an underlying calm, an underlying buoyancy and profundity. No way was I going to be lifted out of the story of my life prematurely. I was in the Lord's hands. This was bedrock certainty for me. But I was not clear about which side of the threshold I would be on in a year. Not my decision. Whichever side I would land on, I would still be in the Lord's hands and continuing my pilgrimage to my true Self.

Our school, Hawthorne Valley, thoughtfully wrapped our house in a blanket of silence. A "Don't call, don't visit" quarantine insulated us. "Everybody is praying for you." At the time, I had no idea to what extent this was true. I began to receive intimations as a blizzard of cards began to come in. There was no keeping my brain tumor discretely a family medical matter. As a teacher in a wonderful school, mine was a most public illness.

My illness was like a pebble dropped in the pool of community. The ripples rayed out in concentric circles to the six directions of a very large pond of relationships. I had not really thought about how many people we were connected to, but, given the life-threatening nature of my illness, the worldwide web of William and Andy's friendships galvanized into a MEDICINE WHEEL, which made these connections clear. Many years ago I had heard a Native American speaker conduct a Medicine Wheel ceremony for Waldorf teachers that reverently recognized the elements, ancestors, creatures, and powers of the six directions. Subsequently, I was instrumental in organizing a festival that included our entire community in a pageant quest. The goal was to travel north, south, east, and west, to the stars above and the earth below to earn the gifts that together could tame the dragon poisoning nature. Now I felt the sacred Medicine Wheel rise again.

Great rings of people of all ages encompassed me. Beyond my family, those holding me in their thoughts and prayers included: the children and parents of my class, the students and parents of the Hawthorne Valley Community, my dear teaching colleagues, my co-workers on the Farm and Visiting Students program, my former students, alumni, members of the Anthroposophical Society, fellow teachers linked through the network of the Association of Waldorf Schools of North America, former students from teacher training programs where I have taught, high school and college friends, the Camphill Community, a congregation in Alabama, the Goddess network, a Native American storyteller, and St. Mary's Catholic Church of Niles, Michigan. Among all these people were Buddhists, Jews, Protestants of all denominations, Meher Baba devotees, Sufis, Muslims, Catholics, Gurdjieffians, devotees of Krishna, agnostics, New Age eclectics, Wiccans, esotericists, astrologers, philosophers, and diverse spiritual seekers. "As many faiths, so many paths." This was a Medicine Wheel with clout. Children's prayers for their teacher are powerful. The meditative strength of this circle could make the blind man see. "Don't give up, pick up your bed and walk!"

I'm a friendly person, interested in people of all kinds and ages. I have dedicated myself to helping build up Hawthorne Valley School. On this life path I have met many people and represented Waldorf education on numerous occasions. Suddenly, spontaneously, in response to my medical crisis there was a great outpouring of good will, prayer, kind thoughts, blessings, and healing energy directed toward me. I would learn that there were people thinking of me dozens, even hundreds of times a day. Like a song you can't shake, William's smiling face (I imagine) would flicker in and out of consciousness of those united in concern for me as they went about their daily work.

In the past, when I had prayerfully tried to support friends in need, I found my poor focus a wavering flame at best. I have since learned that all such flickering thoughts of blessing, all "holding one in the light," whether occurring randomly during the day or tied to specific prayers at a given time, flow into the stream of grace in which we live and breathe and have our being. Our thoughts are real. Hearts' thoughts are prayer.

To be a focal point of such love is an immensely humbling experience. My little "I," hanging in the balance between life and death, was as helpless as a newborn baby. This child was embraced, warmed, beamed on within the cumulative spiritual strength of the coalescing Medicine Wheel. In the breathing in and out of blessing, they gave, I received.

NASA, the Strategic Defense Initiative, or National Security Cybernauts could not detect this evolving, revolving light formation of the Medicine Wheel. It was and is a spiritual force and living presence. It is available to all. Those forming the wheel hold the karmic threads of the light garment of one's life. Each one of us will have a turn in the center. My turn came during surgery.

This is what I saw, heard and felt:

The eternal starry dome bathes us all with infinite light invisibly permeating infinite midnight. A holy, helpless child is encircled by a globe of spirits — hundreds of young and old human beings, wise spirits of the dead, and, behind them, angelic beings who know this infant. All the assembled host

*is spiritually present for his birth in the spiritual world
(what we call death)—or will it be his rebirth in the physical
world? The child feels blissful, surrounded by an ocean of
love. He beams it back from his joyous little heart to the cir-
cumference. This intensifies the love streaming toward him.
The shining faces of all these human and spiritual beings
are visible one by one and as a throng. Each in his own
way is eloquently expressive, filled with spiritual intention,
generous, compassionate, receptive, benevolent. There is
no sorrow or fear, only great good will and warmth. The
Medicine Wheel of those karmically connected to the child
revolves majestically, as beautiful in its geometric structure
as a Mozart symphony or a multi-dimensional stained glass
rose window. The harmony of the stars rings and sings in
the crystal clear spheres of the midnight-blue Empyrean.*

SURGERY

THURSDAY, NOVEMBER 17, 2005. Andy and I are up at 5:00 a.m.
and on the road for Albany Medical Center by 5:45. A meditation
tape is playing. Andy drives. I turn inward.

The beautiful voice of a Harvard psychologist is teaching
me how to relax. Relax. I have been a meditant for thirty years,
with varying degrees of success. The monkey mind, the squirrel
cage of random, unwanted thoughts, can still take me from the
point. But I am not a novice. What do I need tapes for? *Just still
your mind and put this all in the hands of God.* But the tapes, a
gift from a surgeon friend, were in fact very soothing, insightful,
and validated by "scientific research." Who am I to be skeptical
of scientific research? Without it I'd be dead. I am grateful that
science has belatedly found meditation to have salutary effects
on breathing, circulation, the immune system and the whole

mysterious endocrine system, not to mention the heart, soul, and spirit. I was wide open to whatever resources would float my boat. Guided meditation, especially by a trusted guide, is a wonderful support for healing. The attention is directed by a kind voice toward bodily relaxation, soul relaxation, presence of mind, and spiritual readiness. Contrast this with listening to the "Morning Report" of car bombs, refugees, and the "progress" of the war on the radio or one's anxious "roof brain chatter" anticipating surgery. Positive envisioning: successful surgery, successful treatment, joy in life, family love, beautiful memories of a lifetime. Pick a person or a place that makes you happy.... *Breathe.*

Our friend Dr. Branko Furst, the anesthesiologist respected by all, greets us as promised at the door. He had been up all night as a surgical team member for other operations. His warm smile inspired confidence, as much as circumstances would allow. He took Andy and our daughters (who had come in another car) under his wing. I changed into a hospital gown. Much of the time I had an inner mantra going.

This mantra and a few others that were most significant for me, I would come back to again and again in the ensuing days and weeks. It was my custom to recite this verse every day as I walked to school. It had been given by Rudolf Steiner to the first teachers of the Waldorf School:

> Dear God, may it be that I, as far as my personal ambition
> is concerned, quite obliterate myself. Dear Lord, make true
> in me the words of Paul, "Not I, but Christ in me"; that the
> Holy Spirit may hold sway in the teacher.

I will spare you a lengthy theological discussion; meanwhile, the prep squad fishes for my wiggly veins. You say "Allah," he says "Yahweh," she says "Spirit of Humanity," I say "Christ," he says "Ahura Mazdao," she says "Buddha mind," he says "Brahma," she says "Sophia," he says higher "Self," she says "Great Spirit," they say "Hare Krishna," he says "Beloved." Insert the name of the divinity or spiritual guide of your choice here: "I say _____." All these names for the divine, plus the ninety-nine ineffable names of God and Her/His name in all the languages of the world, are mere signposts. Actual spiritual experience occurs in the Holy of Holies of the soul where the spirit flames up like a bright ray of one infinite Sun.

Forgive this interpolation. I am aware, benighted mortal that I am, that the spiritual beings I had the temerity to name are distinct with multifaceted spiritual intentions. My intention is merely to repeat: There are no atheists in the foxholes. When they roll you in for surgery or childbirth or last rites, I know you and your circle of friends will invite the spiritual help that is there for us, as abundant as sunlight to our little, upturned, leaf-like hands.

Let's Roll! I on my physical/spiritual gurney, with a morphine-drip feed, am wheeled down the hall, leaving Andy, Claire, Rosie, and Billie behind. Otto is with his father. I see the ceiling lights, hear the reassuring banter of the technicians...and step into the VOID.

WAKE UP

"IT'S OVER!" As I open my eyes I see Branko's smiling face looking into my eyes. As he tells me "It's over," I'm hearing "It is finished...." Christ's final words on the cross. Branko may be an angel. I need to get my bearings.

I thought no time had passed. In "real time" I had been conveyed to surgery around seven thirty a.m. Another two hours of pre-surgical preparation had taken place. The surgery itself was two and a half hours long. I had been given an anti-inflammatory injection of Decadron to prevent any swelling during and after surgery. I was told that the tumor had been removed. The surgery was a qualified success. The tissue was sent for lab analysis. Malignant (I shudder at the word) or benign (like a generous sovereign)? Much hung in the balance. We would remain in limbo for a few more days on this score. Meanwhile, I would stay under observation in the neurology intensive care unit for one night and the neuro ward a second night.

So much for the earthly plane. Now words fail. They are no substitute for living experience. These faltering phrases will have to suffice as a finger pointing at the moon. Don't mistake the pointing finger for the real thing. During surgery—

I was blown from my body into the cosmos!
The fragments of this profoundly beautiful experience that
    remain in memory I will now try to outline:
I gave myself over to the spiritual beings who protect and
    preserve my life.
I felt supported by a river of grace.
I shed earthly baggage of shame and guilt of my shadow self
    and asked for
 forgiveness.
I felt I had died.
I asked to be made whole or new.
I saw in the starry realm the Medicine Wheel of Life, Light,
    and Love of those many people and spirits who held me
    in their care and keeping.
I saw the Holy Child in the center of that celestial wheel
    who is Every Holy Child, the Christ Child, my baby self,
    my ill self, my true self.
I saw Children of the Future emerging from a rose of light,
    guided one by one by a spiritual being with a gesture of
    blessing. I could not see the features of his face.
I was given to understand that the Spirit of Generosity, the
*   Spirit of Humanity, and other beings had a strong inten-*
*   tion that these Children of the Future be received into*
*   earthly life so they could fulfill their mission—to share*
*   their gifts of will and heart and light with humanity.*

More specifically, my eyes opened to the gifts, capacities, and resolves of this coming generation of Children. I felt that I was given a small role to play toward a convergence of many, many people opening doors for them.

The broad message of this revelation had some very specific directives, connected to my decades of service to the Waldorf philosophy. It was made clear to me in a new way that the Waldorf schools, also known as Rudolf Steiner schools, have a priceless gift that they must share with contemporary culture. Embedded in these schools is an inspiring reverence for the Children of the Future and recognition for the spiritual-earthly collaboration necessary for self-realization. These schools are guardians of the Image of the Human Being. This seed-bearing educational impulse for the future is charged with communicating that loving and living conception of our humanity which leads in time to our becoming more fully human. We are in process, not yet there. However, the inspiring ideals of this education must be made known — *Now*. We in the Waldorf school movement are being asked to take a stand for the integrity of the emerging individual—to stand for the "I," the Child of the Future. No child can be quantified, weighed, or measured by projected outcomes, goals and standards, and mechanistic curricula. We would stand for the freeing of the emerging "I," uniquely expressed by each human being.

It was urgently essential that Steiner education become known and that the doors of Waldorf Schools be opened wider to make room for all those children seeking it.

A blueprint for this happening was given.

I came back to earth and woke up, reborn.

SCROOGE

IT WAS AND STILL is difficult for me to describe what I have written above without "tying rocks to clouds." The act of describing the experience seems inevitably to change it. Maybe you know the Gospel tune, "I said I wasn't going to tell nobody, but I couldn't keep it to myself…what the Lord done done for me." I couldn't talk about the experience rightly and I couldn't not talk about it. I wanted to tell people how I was feeling, what had happened. I was Lazurus emerging from the tomb! I was one of those who, having looked at shadows all his life, is suddenly set free from his chains, to emerge into the clear light of day. All I had assimilated of Steiner's guidance for teachers and all my experience of working with children for thirty years were newly coalesced, illuminated. A hologram of the Image of Humanity had been sealed upon my heart.

Stepping back for a moment, that was Thursday, November 17, 2005. It has taken nearly a year to say what little I have said above. I made some faltering attempts with a few close friends, but the linear nature of language, my own inability to absorb or articulate what had been shown me, and the need to recuperate conspired against my giving over what lived in me. My finer bodies had been blown apart. I had disintegrated. I needed time to reintegrate and find my balance. I was very concerned that the whole vision would fade within three days and I would be left with dim memories or nothing at all of the panorama I am hinting at.

Much of Thursday I was out, floating about the cosmos, reconnecting with my family, sleeping, or simply unconscious. I had continued to receive Decadron, and I was also sedated to sleep off the surgery. The two drugs fought within me for supremacy. When I woke, I felt like Scrooge on Christmas morning!

I was *Alive!* The world was glowing. It was not too late. Three spirits had come, showing Christmas past, Christmas present, and the undetermined Christmas of the Future. Bells were ringing. The erstwhile miser threw open the window to ask what day it was. "Why, it's Christmas morning, Sir." Scrooge inhaled the cold, clear air, like the elixir of life that it is. Giddy with mirth, joy, benevolence, magnanimity, compassion, and good will to humanity all at once, he vows with all his heart selflessly to serve his fellow human beings. He is redeemed, ***Reborn!***

How clear and precious was the light of day. How beautiful were the faces of the people caring for me. I had been given a reprieve, not only a stay of execution, but the door of the prison house had swung open. Scrooge's shackles, forged by selfishness, had fallen away. He was free to do good deeds out of love for humanity — *philanthropy.*

How can I compare myself to Scrooge? He and I share an experience of grace, transformation, and resurrection. *"Die and Become!"* Scrooge and I, and many others, especially cancer patients, through illness have undergone an initiation, a baptism by fire. Cancer as experienced by the patient can go toward either extreme — toward hardening, clinging, closing off, pain, bitterness, or toward expansion, openness, love, walking through the gates of larger life, which are also the gates of death, with Cancer as companion, not as adversary. Cancer can be a gift or nemesis. It depends.

My cancer did not have to do with lack of generosity. I have tended to be generous to a fault in service to my students, school, and community anchored by love of family and inspired by an ideal. But I gave too much of myself away to others. I did not withhold for myself the soul space to fulfill parts of my life's longing. Duty always came before soul-nourishing creative work. Rarely, I could combine the two. As my responsibilities increased, I would take time for committees, administrative work, conflict resolution, and helping others in addition to my primary responsibility to my class. I would not use time for myself. I said "Yes" when I should have said "No." We won't go into the psychology of my personality right now, because the larger picture having to do with *philanthropy* and the Children of the Future commands center stage.

The strange fact is I actually had been Scrooge! As a fifth grader at Westside Elementary School I had urged the class to do a play of *A Christmas Carol.* (This was the second play of my dramatic career since we had performed *Snow White and Rose Red* in first grade. My mother typed it up for us from Grimms'.) I was not satisfied with the dialogue of *A Christmas Carol* as given in our basic reader. There was more to it. I knew. We had a television by this time. It came late, when I was in third grade, because my father wanted to wait until they "got the bugs out of it." (I thank my lucky stars that television came no sooner.) I had seen the 1951 black-and-white version of Scrooge three times by fifth grade. The dialogue, gestures, and facial expression were engraved on my soul. This profound story of rebirth has been with me since my childhood. Now the story had come to life as I threw open the hospital shutters and saw the new day.

Philanthropy

After his rebirth, Scrooge became a philanthropist. He gave his money away, benefiting others. He had everything he needed—life in abundance. Now Scrooge had only one goal and that was bound to his own redemption. He reversed the stream of money from selfish acquisitiveness toward himself to generous benefaction toward others. This became his greatest joy.

In the expansive vision that I received, I, like Scrooge, was allowed a glimpse of the working of karma in my biography past, present, and future. In this panorama of my life I received THE GIFT. The gift was many things simultaneously: the gift of life, the loving gifts of family and friends, the gift of the Medicine Wheel, the gift of my illness, the gift of vision, the gifts the Children of the Future were bringing, the gift of new eyes for nature, the gift of a deeper understanding of being Human. From one day to the next, all that had been before, my persona as teacher, my daily routine, duties, and habits were peeled away. The prospect of death had stripped away all that was nonessential. That refining fire left a vessel empty enough to be filled with THE GIFT. "From you I receive, to you I give, together we share and from this we live." The fullness, loving generosity, the grace of the Giver of All is mirrored back by the recipient's gratitude for the abundant life of creation. The present is the present in all senses of the word. There is the sun and here is a drop of dew. The drop, struck by sunlight, reflects the world around in all its glory. The individual recognizes all the gifts he had taken for granted now comprehended in wholeness. Golden gifts like life, light, and love. This is waking up.

Key to understanding THE GIFT I am attempting to describe is the fact that, by design or coincidence, I had received on behalf of the school the promise of an incredibly generous gift less than two weeks before. This occurred just as I was headed into a steep descent. The same night of the MRI, not yet knowing I had cancer, I called the donor. I was confused in our phone conversation, did I understand correctly? The donor's gift was a challenge, a three-to-one match—three dollars for every new dollar raised. Was I dreaming? Was such generosity possible? The *philanthropy* of the donor was especially directed toward scholarship money becoming available for children who could not otherwise afford our school. The *philanthropist* was the last person outside the school community I talked to before my surgery.

From its inception in 1919, the original Waldorf school and its offspring have carried a social impulse as part of its mission: that the schools be accessible to those who seek them and that they be independent of government control. Here came an unprecedented gift to help us open our doors to more families.

But our little Hawthorne Valley School is just a brush stroke in the mighty panorama of the Children of the Future. They were brimming with the *Spirit of Generosity*. They were inspired to bring their gifts from heaven to earth. It can be said that this is what children, all children, always do. Yes, but there was an especially urgent spiritual intention obvious in this present generation, and no mystery why they were coming *Now*. We needed them. We were in trouble, fragmented, out of balance as a culture. Could it be that our society had forgotten that a child is "a spiritual being in a physical body"? All mechanisms to train children toward high stakes tests, strictly regimented time lines, and quantifiable results were actually damaging the souls of the emerging human beings. "Accountability" of students and teachers to "universal" standards submerged and constricted the miraculous gifts that the children bore beneath encrustations of an unbalanced, inhumane educational system. We are accountable to recognizing the Children of the Future and serving what they actually need to blossom into their creative potential as full human beings. They are not accountable to our misguided attempts at uniformity or to fulfilling economically and politically motivated mandates. Our system has it exactly backward, and nearly everyone has bought into it.

In contrast, *Philanthropy,* love of humankind, recognizes the heart and will forces of children through which the light of thinking catches fire. "Education is not filling a bucket, it is lighting fires."

On the mundane level of our small school, we had a fortunate opportunity to begin to establish a modest scholarship program to begin to open our doors wider. The prototype for the Waldorf schools was subsidized by profits from industry and the personal philanthropy of Emil Molt. Today, though we all support the public school system with our taxes, we must rely on tuition income and gifts to sustain our schools. But here was a very significant gift from an anonymous friend. Could our school begin to lift its head, think creatively, and open itself to receive the abundant generosity of other philanthropists who stood with us for the soul of childhood?

On the spiritual plane, the *Spirit of Generosity* was already moving. The clouds separating heaven from earth are parting. We must be ready to receive these Children of the Future. They offer potent forces of will, love, and light for the healing of our culture. We must find the material and spiritual resources to open our doors and hearts to the Children of the Future. To fail in this is to invite a hardening of the soul, and a loss of spirit.

DARK NIGHT OF THE SOUL

WHEN ICARUS FLEW TOO close to the sun, the wax of his wings melted and he plummeted into the sea.

To prevent seizures during surgery and to stop the swelling and inflammation surrounding the tumor, I was given two powerful drugs, Decadron and Keppra. When a warrior is wounded in battle the entire endocrine system goes on red alert. The adrenal glands instantaneously squirt adrenaline and cortisone into the veins like white lightning. In milliseconds the whole body responds—respiration, heartbeat, circulation, and the muscles. Blood rushes to the vital organs, the senses go hyper-vigilant, and the involuntary reflexes of the brain stem go into hyper drive. Life is at stake: fight, flight, or freeze! Brain surgery in a sterile, cool, controlled environment is far from the battlefield, but a surgical saw to the cranium is for the self-preserving, evolutionarily conditioned reflexes of the reptilian brain indistinguishable from an ax, even if one is mercifully "unconscious." I was in for a crash course in modern pharmacology.

After I was settled in the neuro ward for post-op observation, I could see my family. It had been awful for them to confront the possibility that I might die from the virulent cancer or that I would be permanently brain damaged from the surgery, hardly able to remember things, hardly able to speak. But even these giant specters hid in the shadows. Something only slightly less disturbing arose. I was not myself. As relieved as they were that the surgery was over, it was clear that Dad had gone mad! I was over the edge, talking about some vision. I was a rapper, a speed freak. Why couldn't I just stop and rest and come round normal? The fact was I was desperately concerned that the whole gossamer dream, the vision of THE GIFT, would vanish into thin air. There was precious little time to spit it out, get it down. I was holding a treasure map written in invisible ink. It was on fire, letters appearing for an instant in the flames before they vanished in smoke.

From my urgent perspective, I was trying to share something that had profoundly changed the way I looked at the world and my life. I had a burning sense of purpose on behalf of the Children of the Future. Time was running out. I saw the love and concern in the eyes of Andy and Claire and Rosie. Apparently, I was not coherent. What I was saying sounded fragmented and ranting. They were in the turbo tunnel of my torrent of words, getting windburn. They could not hide their worry that I was exhausting myself when I should be resting from surgery. I tried to throttle down. But I insisted repeatedly that I needed a digital tape recorder to retain the rapidly retreating fragments of THE GIFT. They got me my son-in-law's analog recorder that lasted an hour. How could I begin to record the scope of the live streaming insights flooding in? I was simultaneously tuned to many channels and desperate to preserve all guidance received. "Please get me a digital recorder!"

When alone perhaps I could begin to halt the ebbing of the threshold experience with the recorder in my hand. The directions for its use were microscopic, labyrinthine techno-speak. Thwarted. One menu option sent a shudder through me: DELETE ALL. The ahrimanic gremlins would allow me to gather pitiful bits and bites of digitized cosmic scale Imaginations, which I would attempt to store. Then I would press DELETE ALL by mistake. This fear caused me great anxiety. No one would believe me unless I had "evidence" of what I had received as vision.

Early that evening: "Do you know where you are?" Who speaks out of the blinding light?.... "Albany...Med...." A week before on Dilantin I had responded, "Hawthorne Valley School." Progress. "What is your date of birth?" "October...25...umm 1946." My retrieval system was a little slow on the uptake. "What day is it?" No clue. I was in the twilight zone, and I was flyyyyyyyiiiiiiing on Decadron. This ritual interrogation would recur every hour all night, like a broken record as I tried to figure out who I had been and who I was now. I had gone through the Looking Glass and was not sure which side I was on.

I felt like a peeled rabbit. I had no skin, no protection. I had dis-integrated on the threshold between this world and the next. Humpty Dumpty—my egg-shaped dome, had been blown to smithereens. Now, every sensory stimulus was amplified. I heard multiple conversations in other parts of the ward. I could not lock out the multitude of sounds. Several TVs were on. The decadent exhibitionism and tawdry conflict of the *Jerry Springer Show* came at me with my defenses down. The movement-activated towel dispensers sounded like roaring crowds. Eyelids were no defense against the lights. With clairaudience I was convinced I could hear electricity humming in the lines and lights along with the hissing and ultra-high frequency ringing of my internal systems. Electronic signals, monitoring machines, and call bells randomly went off, each giving a little spurt of adrenalin to my hyper-vigilant nervous system. Electric motors would intermittently whir to raise or lower a bed or swing a mechanical arm into place. The continuous bombardment of sound felt intentionally devised to prevent sleep. I was being kept awake on purpose. "What's your name? Do you know where you are? What is your date of birth? Now I'm going to shine a light into your eyes." The intrusive light invades the optic nerve and frightens the bats in my belfry. The drill was repeated every hour.

The nurse told me not to move because of my head bandage. I took it literally and froze in a knotted position for an interminable period. Time crawled, then stopped dead. This Dark Night of the Soul would be eternal. The Shadow of Death was waiting in the wings. There would be no day. No exit. No resurrection. I was already in Purgatory, part of a sensory overload experiment. I was paranoid that I would be kept in constant wakefulness. They would not let me go home. The room and rounds were designed not to let patients slip into the healing waters of sedated oblivion. The drill was to rouse them and monitor them to keep them here and not let them slip over the edge into the Never Never Land of a coma.

I have never longed for unconsciousness so intensely. I wanted to be entombed, *enwombed* in total darkness, in total silence. If only I could reintegrate in a subterranean crypt where I could be consoled and refreshed in a haven of peace, and get myself together. I began to redesign in my overactive mind the neuro ward as it should be for human beings with walls of color, soft celestial music, the wash of the sea. Lazurus-like neophytes in padded sarcophagi slept the temple sleep in silent, underground caverns in my hospital of the future. Hierophant nurses, the Therapeutae, ministered to their patients' needs in body, soul, and spirit as healing streams of peace and light washed the weariness and fear from their blood and bones.

Speaking softly into the recorder, doubting whether anything was being stored, I began to monitor the number of sounds per minute to pass the time, since sleep was impossible. I understood why sleep deprivation is a form of torture and how it leads to a disintegration of the personality.

The night nurse worked on the accumulated paperwork from the day. The necessary act of stapling papers together sent the amplified sound straight through me. I was being stapled alive. By perhaps two a.m. I so longed for oblivion that I asked to be knocked out. I was given Ambien. I entered a Twilight Zone where Ambien and Decadron could duke it out over my wounded body and soul.

Later I discovered that there is an epidemic of sleeplessness in our land. Ambien and Lunesta have annual gross sales of about 1.5 billion annually, with around fifty million prescriptions each year for sleep aids. That is the downer side of the spectrum. Big pharma rakes it in. But why is it people's sleep is so disturbed that this avalanche of pharmaceuticals is needed? As I expressed to one of my nurses my reluctance to put so many chemicals in my body, she commented matter-of-factly, but out of earshot of those who might think differently, "We are a nation of drug addicts."

GUARDIAN ANGELS

PRIOR TO THE RESPITE of Ambien, I had several brief but intensely meaningful exchanges with members of the nursing staff who came to check on me. Who are these angels of mercy who keep vigil through the night and bring encouragement and compassionate care by day? Not only was my cranium surgically opened, but my revivified heart could now see that these people were sisters and brothers of mercy. They treated every patient and their concerned family members with respect, empathy, and understanding.

Given the hospital setting and my life-threatening situation, the words of Christ (Matthew 25) helped me see the people caring for me in a most profound light:

> Then shall the King say unto them on his right hand, Come, ye blessed of my Father, inherit the kingdom prepared for you from the foundation of the world: For I was hungry and ye gave me meat: I was thirsty, and ye gave me drink: I was a stranger, and ye took me in: Naked, and ye clothed me: I was sick, and ye visited me: I was in prison, and ye came unto me.
>
> Then shall the righteous answer him, saying, Lord, when saw we thee hungry, and fed thee? Or thirsty, and gave thee drink? When saw we thee a stranger and took thee in? Or naked, and clothed thee? Or when saw we thee sick, or in prison, and came unto thee?
>
> And the King shall answer and say unto them, Verily I say unto you, Inasmuch as ye have done it unto one of the least of these my brethren, ye have done it unto me.

The Family of Humanity was well represented by these active caregivers: a slight, shy Vietnamese woman; a hip, hilarious African-American male nurse; an expatriate Russian practical nurse; a graceful Filipina night nurse; an outgoing Evangelical San Salvadorian orderly, a young Indian intern, a veteran registered nurse ward supervisor ("She Who Wears the Pin"). She had returned to the trenches from the ranks of administration because this is where the person-to-person action is. There were others who flitted in and out of my range of vision, but these five diverse individuals shone with particular radiance. The combined effects of the surgery, the Decadron, my unbounded gratitude for being alive, the Scrooge-like awakening, and the continuing streaming of the super-sensible Medicine Wheel, were like an effervescent elixir—Aqua Vita. I overflowed with respect for my benefactors and was completely dependent upon their kindness and expertise. Their vitality, therapeutic will, and proactive insight was of continual service to others. These heroes and heroines are placed among us exactly where needed most. I have no reason to doubt that I was cared for by angels in human garb.

So-called reality had undergone a radical realignment. I wondered what sort of people find their fulfillment in continually helping others? People of profound good will. Unlike the capitalist system of enlightened self-interest, these souls applied the opposite principle—enlightened selflessness. "Thy will be done, *on earth* as it is in heaven." In the economy of the healing arts, their surplus of energy was generously given to those with waning forces. They were power generators in the worldwide grid of human needs. Strangely, the more they gave, the more they had to give. Whom did they serve? The one closest, then the one next on their perpetual rounds.

I don't mean to imply there aren't overworked medical staff dragging around, already carrying their share of life's burdens. But somehow they have the inner resources to take on the additional load of the sick, weary, and weak. I was privileged by the blessing of my illness to look into the eyes of authentic, strong, salt-of-the-earth human beings on the front line of human suffering. "What ails thee, brother?" They know why they are here, and they know what they are doing. There is no gap between seeing and acting. They are plugged into the self-renewing power supply of healing will.

It was all completely matter-of-fact. I imagine a pep talk from a chorus of my caregivers: "You wanted a body. Now let's deal with it. Vomit, excrement, blood, viscera, that's OK. We've got mops, we've got sponges. That's part of having a body. Ain't no stain we can't clean. We will bathe you, we will feed you, whether you are skin and bones or round like a baby. Bring it on. There is nothing you can show me —no wound, sore, burn, fracture, scab, exudation, pustule, tumor, ulcer, inflammation, secretion, excretion, or trauma that I have not seen before. Fear not. Nothing can turn me away. I am your sister-brother and I am here for you."

Scrooge takes note. This is again *philanthropy*, love of humanity. The currency is care, *charitas*, charity. This is the breathing heart of giving and receiving. I was sick and you cared for me. How grateful I am to receive your kind help.

Small thing. During the night I had heard the simple phrase, "Thank you," repeated so many times. "Thank you" was echoing down the wards and around the world in all languages. Giving a helping hand—acknowledging the gift of service. Two sides of the same coin:

"Thank you"— "You're welcome."
"Call if you need me"— "Thank you."
"That feels better, thanks"— "Glad to help."
"Thanks for the juice"— "Anytime."
"Can I get you anything?"— "Thanks for the extra pillow."
"Let me know if I can help"— "Thanks, I will."

This simplest human transaction, reenacted innumerable times a day, is the universal gesture of human kindness.

> From you I receive,
> To you I give,
> Together we share
> And from this we live.

I had known for years in the abstract that "think" and "thank" grew from the same root. I knew also that grace, *gratis*, and gratitude were cognate with one another. But now, in a state of grace, at least temporarily, I could feel the warm humanity standing within the exchanges I could overhear, the empathetic recognition of one another's needs and generosities. The offering hand and the open hand touching, forming the circle of giving and receiving. A child receives a small gift. "Don't forget to say, 'Thank you,'" says an infinite chorus of Mothers through the ages. The child shyly looks at her benefactor and says, "Thank you." "You are welcome. It's my pleasure." This generous reciprocity, so commonplace as to be hardly noticed, is the foundation of community. You can depend on the time-honored power of "Thanks." Thanksgiving was in the air!

In this same vein, a dozen years ago I had a sudden flash of intuition. I know it was important because I remember exactly my location and the slant of light as I was leaning against the kitchen counter in Niles, Michigan. I have no idea what brought on the Sudden Revelation: "Why are we here?" I wondered, and the answer came. *"We are fountains of joy and love!"*

Who was speaking in my mind?

Don't misunderstand those words as clichéd, sentimental, greeting-card drivel. They are simple words filled with life. Just take a drink from that inexhaustible spring and see what you can do then. Thank you hospital caregivers, teachers of kindness.

SHADOW AND DAYLIGHT

THE DARK NIGHT OF the Soul is a passage through the Valley of the Shadow of Death. "Where there is great light, there is great shadow." What I had experienced as a resurrection, waking to the fullness of life, and a reprieve from death was bound to its opposite: a Night Journey too intense at the time for me to speak about.

According to ancient rituals of initiation, one of the inevitable steps toward awakening to consciousness of the spiritual world was dismemberment; the lower self had to die before the higher self could be born. Two difficult nights from nightfall till dawn were part of my death process. "Dissolution," "disintegration," and "dismemberment" are too abstract for what I am referring to. Let me give a picture: Open your art history book to Heironymous Bosch; examine the goads, the fires, the demons, the implements of torture, the chaos and fear, the sores, the animal heads on human bodies, the dance of death. Imagine that you are no mere onlooker, but stripped and flogged; you have been sucked into the nightmare vortex and abandoned all hope. This demonic realm confronts you with the grotesque, bizarre emanations of the lower self. You lose yourself in the astral enticements and torments of living hell until its refining fires have purged away the dross. When the molten gold of the sun's tears alone remains, the alchemical process of transformation is complete.

I was not swept into the maelstrom. Whoever was guiding my little boat managed to steer between Scylla and Charybdis. My helpers were there to cut off the hydra's heads of my once rampantly proliferating glioblastoma multiforme and cauterize the stumps. I felt protected. Undeniably my senses were too open, as described earlier, and a part of me was "flayed" by sensory overload. But I had fully entrusted myself to the guidance and guardianship of the spiritual world to see me through. My fear of death in this world was obliterated by the conviction that I had already died and mysteriously, joyfully was called back to take care of unfinished business. To receive the grace of this reprieve I had to give up my Shadow. In my case, the prospect of death allowed me to drop some of the burden of my karmic baggage and lighten my load. There is a lot more to do. There was a cleansing, purging process under the sign of cancer that now allows me to take further steps along my healing journey. To do this I must find the resolve.

I don't want to tell you about my Shadow. The shame is too great. It is a skeleton in the closet, too painful to acknowledge. It is a weight, a burden of guilt, a feeling of unworthiness. Behind my mask, I'm no good. I have failed myself, my possibilities of becoming. I have betrayed the trust placed in me at birth to seek my star. Having fallen far short of my humanity, I must keep the beast, the truth, hidden and chained.

Does this resonate with anyone out there? But there is one who knows and accepts what I choose not to share. This generous spirit is my witness and guide. This is the gentle brother, "friend of my heart." This is he who sees me as I am and would lead me in my becoming. I am the prodigal son who has wasted his inheritance. I am Jonah, fleeing God and the path set for me, swallowed up in the belly of the whale. But One comes bearing the healing cup of forgiveness. He frees me from the chains that bind me to my Shadow and leads me into larger life.

A decade ago, a friend was struggling with AIDS. In his final year, I sent him a print of a painting by Holman Hunt. I was wrestling with my Shadow at the time I encountered the painting, as I have many times since. The work is *The Light of the World* from Keble College, Oxford. With cosmic irony, the light illuminating it went out as I was looking on. Now, since I have jettisoned baggage I had been carrying, the picture has resurfaced. The light has come back on. I had forgotten that my friend's mother had returned it to me at his death. During recovery from surgery, I found it in my attic. Now it's by my bed, the first thing I see when I wake up. It is a night scene. There are faint stars and a bat. A seldom-used door is overgrown with dried weeds. Christ, his face faintly illumined by the lantern he holds, knocks on the door. The inscription reads:

> Behold I stand at the door and knock.
> If any man hear my voice and open the door
> I will come in to him
> And will sup with him
> *And he with me.*
> Open the door if you would receive the Guest.

On my release from the hospital, as I reviewed my life through papers and photos filed away, a copy of the poem I wrote for my friend, dead for ten years, also resurfaced for the occasion of my return, having come through a Dark Night into daylight.

TRAVELING LIGHT

I have walked the sleeping earth,
Plunged in the restless sea,
Weathered alone mountain storms,
Known stars' serenity;

Run the rage of rivers,
Wandered canyons deep,
Sought peace in forest temples,
Scaled rock backbone steep;

Quenched thirst's fire in mountain springs,
Crossed the desolate dunes,
Stone-still become the sunset
And drifted with the moon;

Understood birds' twilight song,
Named ten thousand things,
Descended into shadow,
Risen on eagle's wings.

Now I vow a pilgrimage,
I intend to travel light,
I will explore, by myself,
Striding day and night

A path through the wilderness
Few have found before,
Beyond land's known horizon
To the sacred door—

Where my brother, guide, and friend,
Calls lovingly for me,
Whose healing hand purifies
And sets my spirit free

To cross with him fear's abyss,
To pass with him cold night,

Till his still voice bids me wake
To see sun's morning light

With which sorrow is transformed,
Through which death to life is born,
In whom I see who I am
On the way that has no end.

PICK UP YOUR BED AND WALK

BREAKFAST! COFFEE! LIFE! LOUIS, the Salvadoran orderly, delivers breakfast with a sunshine smile that melts away the Shadow of Death. To me Louis is a saint, a wise man camouflaged in hospital scrubs, one of those Children of the Future who came down to earth knowing exactly what was needed: relieve the burdened, feed the hungry, minister to the sick, visit the imprisoned, help the poor. To me, with heart cracked open, Louis was a Sun Hero, radiating healing humor, good will, and compassion. I needed to know the source of his energy. He blessed his dear departed mother. He knew she was still with him. She had taught him always to be helpful to those in need. He thanked God for the blessing of his life and the energy to serve others. He had always been like this, wanting to help wherever help was needed. "That's the way God made me. It makes me happy to do things for people." No wonder everybody loved him. He never held back. There is joy in his work, in all his actions. It streams out of the center of his heart and face. When he woke in the morning, he prayed for EVERYONE, not just those whom he served in the hospital. He takes the refreshment of the night and expends it all on the selfless actions of the day willingly, giving himself away like sunlight. When he retired in the evening, he put his things in order, said his prayers, and went to bed, receiving his day's wages in the bliss of deep sleep.

Louis lives in the Now. You had to be ready to respond to whatever comes. You never knew when or whether your time was up. "If the Lord says, 'Louis, it's time to go.' I go! Right now, if I am called, I go!" I told him, "You, you're not going anywhere. You have work to do." It was clear to me that Louis was plugged into a higher channel. Being with Louis was communion. He was radiant with healing will. St. Francis's prayer is Louis's prayer:

> Lord, make me an instrument of your peace.
> Where there is hatred, let me sow love;
> where there is injury, pardon;
> where there is doubt, faith;
> where there is despair, hope;
> where there is darkness, light;
> and where there is sadness, joy.
>
> O Divine Master, grant that I may not so much seek to
>   be consoled as to console;
> to be understood as to understand;
> to be loved as to love;
> for it is in giving that we receive;
> it is in pardoning that we are pardoned;
> and it is in dying that we are born to eternal life.

"Don't let your coffee get cold." Louis brought me much more than breakfast. He showed the power of will and heart forces that I recognized in the coming generation, those whom I had seen eager to come to earth: the Children of the Future.

I geared up to return to life. Andy would pick me up this very afternoon. My supersonic hearing detected a conversation between the head nurse and my doctors twenty feet away. "Is he ready to go home? He's had an extreme reaction to his medication; perhaps we should keep him under observation for another day?" This could not be happening! If I made a scene about how desperate I was to get to home sweet home, it would only confirm suspicions that I was having a psychotic reaction to my medication and was delusional. My fate hung in precarious balance. Dr.

German assured the nurse that I would be fine, resting at home. Release was at hand!

I took a warm shower assisted by a nurse's aid. The motif of the miraculous in the everyday extended to the shower: Sun, clouds, rain, water of Adirondack lakes, fire, boilers, pipes, soap, my body—freshly baptized. Going home.

I did a little physical therapy, as they made sure that I could handle the normal functions of daily life. I was not to lift anything weighing more than five pounds until the six-inch incision in my skull healed. I would not drive until further notice, a proscription that lasted over five months.

There was Andy! Van, a Vietnamese nurse's aid, rolled me to the front door. While Andy got the car, Van and I talked. Her voice was musical and soothing. She confided that she had been teased as a young child about singing, a cutting remark from an older sister, so she had considerately stopped. How many of us are carrying similar wounds? But my opened ears could hear the music of her soul. I urged her to take up singing again. I could see that with a little encouragement this could be freed in her and become a treasure rather than a shame. She brightened at my interest and encouragement. The next months would be filled with such small encounters. My new lease on life allowed me to intuit hidden gifts, fears, and aspirations in those I met. People opened up to me. I would hang a shingle outside my door that said, "Listener." People would come to me, I imagined, and the warm human interest of my listening would allow them to see themselves in a new and higher light, freeing creative powers long buried.

The automatic doors opened...then a hunter who had been shot in the face or eye walked in with blood streaming down. He was wearing full camouflage and combat boots. He walked stoically on his own steam, not even holding a rag to the head wound. Back in the real world. I needed to get to the sanctuary of home.

As we drove I could not take my eyes off the passing trees. In my altered state, or should I say "altared" state, the trees seemed to me like neurons rising from a conscious earth as my brain cells rose from the glial mass, the white matter of the brain. All these living, reaching, ramifying branches were receiving the news of the universe from all directions. The fifteen trillion neurons of my brain were mirrored in the macrocosmic network of the arboreal forests. This inconceivably immense forest cover raised up green leaves of all denominations perennially in salutation to the sun. The dead leaves had already fallen to molder on the forest floor until they become the soil of new life, rising again as sap, bud, and leaf. The veins of each leaf, carrying the waters of life, nourished the chlorophyll so closely resembling our blood. Each leaf reflected in miniature the form of the Mother Tree. Springing and Falling forever.

At sunset we came into Hawthorne Valley. The orange-gold of the setting sun streamed across the green fields of home. Every inch on Hawthorne Valley Farm was precious to me from years of walking the land. It was inexpressibly beautiful at this moment. The first person we saw was our dear neighbor, Nicole, welcoming us back from the hospital. She took my hand. She is a trained nurse. She offered me foot massages to help me sleep. Her face was gold in the sunlight, her eyes brimming with compassion for my condition. As we pulled away, she called out, "Don't forget me. I am your neighbor."

In the weeks ahead, Nicole was a frequent visitor at our house. What a tender mercy a foot massage is. The ecstasy of nerves, the happy capillaries, the silken skin, the piggie toes, the articulate bones, the longing ligaments! Feet, humble servants, you who carry us over the body of the earth, you whom I have forgotten till now, you who live so far away and ask for so little, receive now full gratitude for all you do. Nicole applies the magic of healing hands, rhythmically caressing calves, ankles, feet and toes with blackthorn oil. Enlivened blood dances back to the sun of the heart. Etheric forces lap like leafy fire through my body. The laying on of hands is an act of grace. Christ washed the feet of his disciples. "As you do unto one of these, the least of my brethren, you do so unto me." May I learn to be as generous as my good neighbor? Feet, I feel you.

THANKSGIVING

NOVEMBER 20, 2005. HOME! I was in my sanctuary. Dear friends had provided a smoked turkey, with the incredible brand name of "Willie Bird." I lit the hearth-heart fire in what would become an unfailing daily ritual. After the antiseptic, colorless environment of the hospital, the familiar furnishing and atmosphere of home were vibrant with color and coziness. Objects long taken for granted emanated meaning and memories in the security of sacred space. Home was the antidote to the radical changes in our life, that feeling of being on a stormy sea. Here in the sanctuary, the love of family, the calmness of cooking, the blessings over the meal, the delicious food, the ritual washing of the dishes, peacefully enjoying the dancing flames, created such a feeling of well-being, of peace, that no man could ask for more. I was alive. Andy, my soul mate, was with me. Family and friends surrounded me. I had come through the fire. A continuous song of praise and thanksgiving welled up in me. "…My cup runneth over. Surely goodness and mercy shall follow me all the days of my life and I shall dwell in the house of the Lord forever."

FROM MY JOURNAL

Thanksgiving was perfect for family harmony. We realize we are all held in the circle of friendships as surely as we are held in the Medicine Wheel enveloping all of us. This reverberating sphere holds a singular being, a beloved friend, in a vast circle of human connections. He is held lovingly, protected by all good thoughts.

It had snowed overnight. The world was white. Morning Feng-shui was again exquisite. As soon as I awoke, there was a knock at the door. It was Ingo! "I promised you a mousse when you came back from the hospital. Here it is." He gave me a perfect dessert: radiating star form of chocolate on the surface of the mousse with a raspberry on each ray. Ingo's desserts have a reputation. This one was for me. No one can imagine my delight. This warm act of friendship touched me to the core. I knew the mousse had been delayed by a day. Dr. Hertle, Ingo's wife of twenty years and our primary-care physician, had hit black ice on the way back from Camphill Village where she puts in fourteen- to sixteen-hour days. She rolled, the car totaled. They do not need this. They are housing a woman whose husband tragically died a month ago. Now this. Thank you Lord, for sparing my doctor.

Thank you, Ingo, for your friendship." We hug good-bye. This is going to be a great day!

The patient attended to the details of his duties with Be-Here-Now attention. Thanksgiving preparations under the leadership of Andy would be attended to harmoniously in the peaceful rhythm of the enduring rituals of the great Feast. I would have a cameo role in vacuuming the sacred precincts and the preparation of the endive and salmon appetizer. The Great Mother made the corn bread stuffing early. I got to polish the dining room table. It had belonged to my grandparents who were born in the late 1800s. Polishing it was like being with them all over again, "Over the river and through the woods to grandmother's house we go...." I was in the presence of my ancestors and they in me. Behold the altar of the feast.

In the late afternoon Rosie and Billy, Claire, Josh, and Otto arrived with a spectrum of delicacies. Josh and Andy continued their culinary artistry, secrets of gravies and sauces, in the kitchen. Claire and Rosie saw to the setting of the table with wedding china and silver while I played with Otto before the fire. It would have been festive enough as a family circle to share this wonderful meal together, featuring the succulent "Willie Bird," simply, but the ritual was a festival of Life!

Family, communion, love, wedding of Cana, Passover, the Last Supper, Rebirthday, Lazurus, the Prodigal Son, Easter Morning, Thanksgiving all merged into one. Think. Thank. Pray. Praise.

Home. The colors and savor of the food, the shining silver, the glowing gold candles, the white Damask cloth, the flowers, the blessings, the earthy green beans, cornmeal dressing, squash risotto, pumpkin pie, mixed greens salad, hearty appetite, the hilarity, nostalgia, hopes, our joy in one another—thank you Lord for the day Thou hast made.

❧

My sudden departure from Hawthorne Valley School was a great shock for everyone. The children I taught, their parents, the circle of colleagues, the parent body, and wider circles. No one knew how I was doing, what the surgery uncovered, what my prognosis was, what the future held, whether I would return to teaching. When could people visit?

Even though Andy and I knew little about the outcome of the surgery, prescribed treatment, therapeutic options, financial implications, and life-changing nature of the illness, I strongly felt the urge to communicate with my community to thank everyone for their prayerful support and to share what little we knew. I began to write open "Letters from William," which were sent to my colleagues and school parents and were available at the Farm Store.

November 22, 2005
Dear Friends and Colleagues,

What would you do if you received the tremendous outpouring of love that rose like the West Wind and came my direction? I reflect it back to you, and say with a big smile on my face, "Thank you from the center of my heart."

My family thanks you with me for your 10,000 kindnesses, prayers, offers of help, and practical goodness. Thank you especially for the great Prayer Wheel. We are friends. We are community. All our relatives are here! Thanksgiving!

In honor of your gift of love to me there is a gift I make—my gift of love for you. These gifts are each other's mirror. And we realize that *everyone* is in the sunlight, including William, who feels, "God, I love this place. Look how people treat you when you need a friend! Anyone would do anything, day or night, to help out!"

Let us all pass through this circle—the Medicine Wheel, the loving embrace of our friends. When the chips are down, the Food Chain starts!

Love to each of us from each of us (You do the geometry),

> Love, Life, Light!
> Your friend,
> William

PROTECTION

I have been given a gift. I am Scrooge reborn. (I know it's hard to think of me that way.) I am living in silence and growing in thankfulness in my heart and home. We will find time to share. But right now, I am keeping to a peaceful center. Oh, the beauty of Thanksgiving.

❧

I emailed this Thanksgiving prayer to the fourth-grade families to be read at their family gatherings:

> **Thank you,** *dear friends and family, for holding me with such kindness in your heart.*
>
> **Thank you,** *dear earth, for the gift of this food we have prepared from your body. We will eat it with reverence and delight.*
>
> **Thank you,** *water pure that flows in the ocean, falls in rain and snow, flows through our bodies, and helps us clean the dishes.*
>
> **Thank you,** *mantle of air that whirls over the globe, for being the breath inside and outside our bodies, that keeps us awake, refreshes us in sleep, and keeps life moving.*
>
> **Thank you,** *hearth fire—heart fire—sun within, bright sun without—for giving us your warmth.*

Thank you, *Mother of the Family, for all you do. We would not be here without your love for us.*
Thank you, *Father of the Family, for your virtue, which gives strength for the good of all.*
Thank you, *unknown friend, for being here with us today while we enjoy life together.*
Let us remember those in need. May we find ways that they too may share in the feast in the Family of Man.
Amen, Shalom, Salem, Shanti, Peace, Love, Light, Life, L'Chaim.
Blessings on our meal. Happy Thanksgiving.

When the blessing had been read in several festive corners of the county, it trickled back to me that several adults and children had the strong feeling that I was present, with them at the feast. Who knows?

My first night back in my own bed, I offered my deepest thanks to the "Friend of my heart":

> Dear Lord, you led me
> Through the gates of death
> Into the light of larger life.
> May I serve you with every breath
> As you take me to my rest.

On Sunday morning after Thanksgiving, a great, gentle peacefulness, settled over the landscape. By "Thanksgiving" I don't mean just the holiday bearing that name; I mean THANKSGIVING, NOW, the continuously arising conscious thankfulness for the gift of life. My mood and the mood of the day are captured in my journal entry, written as I soaked it all in from my porch:

Let me make clear for myself the peaceful yet overflowing abundance I am in.

Warm, benevolent light is all around me. My body is relaxed, seated, would it be exaggeration to say, "I am enthroned"? The sky is as blue as the veil of the Madonna. I feel particularly close to her today. I have received Mother's

Mercy, which I so sorely needed. I've been trying to go it alone for too long. She took me in and lifted me up in her loving arms. Then we could look into each other's eyes and find out how it is with one another and play peek-a-boo. Then she put me back on my feet—little man—to do my work. I receive her caress, her help, her body, her warmth, her sacrifice, her joy in me, her teaching of me, her listening to me, her telling me stories, her giving me food, her holding my hand, her nursing me when I am ill, soothing me when I am sad, calming me when I am angry, helping me in a thousand ways a day, like tying my shoes. Her fingers can fix anything. She is very patient and kind to everyone—little children and old people and animals. And she has many friends among all women because they understand each other, all having the mother's heart and the mother's body. I revere you, my Mother. I will be your good son. How often I would have given up without your help. Only your heart is big enough, generous enough to receive my pain, my fear, my anger, my sorrow. I ask for your forgiveness, dear Mother. I ask your grace, dear Mother, and, most of all, I ask for your heart—heart of love. Your robe, the blue mantle of the breath of life surrounds us. Beneath your feet and on each hand all fruitfulness appears. As you gaze into my open face, know how much I love you.

LETTERS FROM WILLIAM

I FELT GRATEFUL FOR THE isolation and sanctuary of home as I recuperated from surgery. Andy and I had time and space to begin to process the implications of my illness, though we would not have a prognosis for at least a week.

I was concerned that there were a lot of people in limbo, as were we, who were anxious to learn how I was faring and how serious my illness was. I felt called upon to get the word out, quash unsubstantiated rumors, and gratefully acknowledge the fact and the *experience* of the Medicine Wheel of friends' prayers. Meanwhile, down at the Farm Store, the hub of Hawthorne Valley activity, my son-in-law Josh was getting windburn at his post behind the cash register, responding to people's questions about me. To shield him in some small degree and to try to answer questions simultaneously rather than sequentially, I decided to share what little we knew:

Dear Community,

THANK YOU FOR A VERY HAPPY THANKSGIVING WITH MY FAMILY.

How warmly you are carrying our family. How lovingly you are carrying me. My family sends its deepest Thanks.

We want to let you know we had the best Thanksgiving we have ever had. We were so happy to be together!

There is no ringing phone. I feel better, younger than I have for years. I am home. I am being knit back together. Andy, Claire, Rosie, Josh and Billy have observed my healing process and are very encouraged. My doctors and therapists are encouraged and encouraging. The whole experience for me is filled with grace.

> *The older I get*
> *The younger I grow,*
> *Surrounded by the people I know.*

We put our heads together in family council to determine how best to communicate with you. This is what we decided: We realize the integrity of our healing requires both *openness and protection*. We have chosen to distribute this open letter to all of you in sealed envelopes to each of you.

THE LETTER FROM WILLIAM

William had miraculously successful brain surgery, returning home in two and a half days. What next? You may want to pick a selection of personal responses from the list below:

1. Angelic hosts are not going to let William be taken away from us. He has unfinished business.
2. If William goes, I go.
3. He needs my permission.
4. There is no better place than here.
5. Offer him incentives to stay.
6. Pull celestial strings, talk with people at the top, speak directly to God or the deity of the denomination of your choice (unless you have not been able to find one yet).
7. Stay inwardly open.
8. Talk with family members (BAD IDEA).
9. Talk with William directly (Forbidden. He is Hermetically sealed in his cocoon according to the strictures of the Therapeutae).
10. William who?
11. Surrender desire for a specific outcome.
12. Curse the darkness on his behalf.
13. Go about one's business cheerfully.
14. Go about one's business grumpily.
15. Drop all business.
16. Puzzle over duality.
17. Keep to the Tao.
18. Wait and see.
19. Fuggedaboudit.

Of these diverse outcomes, the toughest for me to hold is "Wait and see."

I refuse. I am not waiting, and I am already seeing. I see you. I *know* what you are doing for me. The Medicine Wheel of your good thoughts and prayers is ringing all around me.

Thank you. Thank you. Thank you. We just had the best Thanksgiving of our lives.

By coincidence, if you believe in that nonsense, I looked on the back of my mirror when I returned from the hospital. A prescient friend had written there many years ago this beautiful Spanish proverb: "In living, our true hearts say 'Yes' to courage and 'No' to fear."

All is well. Your friend,
William

P.S. When Andy and I know what's up on the material plane, based on the expert council of the doctors treating me, Andy and I will follow the prescribed next steps on my therapeutic path.

Meanwhile drink the elixir: Life – L'Chaim!

COMMUNITY — COMMUNION

On November 29, Andy and I spoke with Dr. German, the neurosurgeon who had performed the "resection" operation. He gave it to us straight. The tumor was malignant. We learned that more than half of those who harbor phase IV glioblastoma multiforme die within a year.... (Don't sugar-coat it, Doc). The surgery successfully removed eighty percent of the tumor. Recurrence was a distinct possibility at the site of the resection and really anywhere tendrils had reached within the brain cavity. Dr. Susan Weaver would supervise the allopathic treatment. Standard treatment would include thirty-three doses of radiation, guided by Dr. Kim, and twelve months of chemotherapy using Temodar. This relatively new treatment had become standard procedure for this cancer within the last few years. We would soon learn that it made no grand claims. Statistically it could prolong the survivor's life an average of 1.3 years after surgery. We were all jockeying for that position. I asked some of my many questions. Andy did the same. These treatments would begin as soon as possible. I asked, "What would you think about our taking a trip to Italy?" (Subtext: after my treatments, in the time still allotted to me). "After your radiation treatment, if you feel well enough, take the opportunity." (Subtext: this is likely your last trip, so do whatever you want to do right now.)

I followed up this visit with another open letter to the community.

LETTER FROM WILLIAM

November 30, 2005
Dear Community Members,

Thank you for your powerful prayers. I feel your positive support all around me.

Yesterday Andy and I went to visit Dr. German (you know you are in good hands). We had a very constructive conversation regarding ongoing therapeutic protocol. After speaking with Dr. Hertle, our dear friend who is guiding my therapy, we will continue to research ongoing therapeutic possibilities with two specialists in Albany and a circle of professional alternative therapists. Many of these skilled practitioners are also personal friends. Outside of a metropolitan center, where else you could find such a therapeutic environment?

It has been brought home with stunning clarity that little ole me, among countless fellow travelers, is being included in the prayers of congregations in Alabama, Goddess circles, the Waldorf school movement, the Hawthorne Valley network, the prayers of little children, our extended family, our Tibetan friends, and St. Mary's Catholic Church of Niles, Michigan, in addition to the circle of friends we see from our perch on Fern Hill. This is big time. No wonder I feel so well.

How is it that I feel years younger and more myself while convalescing from brain surgery? My life has changed. My family and I are processing the ramifications of our new situation as they unfold. We appreciate your giving us the space to do our homework. It is not given to us to know exactly where things stand. We are on a steep learning curve and working methodically to discover what therapies best fit my case. Two things we know for sure: I feel ten years younger and well-loved by all of you.

The Food Chain has begun. It starts with old friends among the faculty, will extend to parents in my class, and then will include parents and friends who sign on. Obesity is the next challenge, and returning dishes without mixing them up.

I won't be having a string of visitors to the house. It is rest time. I will probably see two visitors a day maximum, one of them at Food Chain time. That means the chance to sit and talk about the great themes of life and death will be conducted at an extremely leisurely pace over a couple of months no matter how closely we are personally connected. I am a gregarious person in seclusion. My therapeutic schedule is sacrosanct. I will not be giving a public lecture where I could see you all at once titled: "There and Back Again: William's Quest." My lips for now are sealed in self-restraint.

I have made a firm resolve to become a better listener. You thought I was OK in listening before? But now I hear with full attention. So we are in a paradoxical situation: my healing requires sanctuary, and your loving concern deserves to be met with open clarity.

There is a solution. Instead of speaking with one person after another, we have found a way that I can hear your unique voice. Not on the phone, yet not face to face. You speak, I listen.

To "speak," if you wish, take an index card from Josh at the Farm Store. Condense your words of wisdom or insight into a kernel. Commit this to the card in the moment. Drop it in my makeshift mailbox. This Air Mail will be wafted up to my aerie like a leaf on the wind. These words are read by me with recognition for they who live behind the runes: you. I hear exactly what I need to hear. You offer. I receive.

❧

Sample conversation re-enacted in the Farm Store daily: "Josh, how is he doing? I mean really." "He's doing great. I have never seen him so...present." "Can you say anything about what William might be facing medically?" "No, we haven't had time to discuss that as a family. He is not talking about his therapeutic status or post-operation procedures. They are being researched with experts. It would not surprise me if he put it all in a newsletter, but I don't think Andy and Claire would let him. He is a very open kind of guy. I mean, like, OPEN. He told me to tell you that if you want to 'speak' with him, just take one of these index cards. Look inside yourself and jot down a note. Whatever comes to you in the act of writing it down lights up in William when he reads it. It can be short. Like a fortune cookie, like a message in a bottle. Have a nice day."

That's the news from Fern Hill,

Love to you all,
William

❧

This radical shift in how I had imagined my life unfolding would shake all our assumptions. All those children, parents, and colleagues, expecting my imminent return after a modest leave of absence, needed to know that was not in the cards. I knew my fourth grade students were in good hands. The council of teachers had them foremost in mind, and Candace Christiansen was there for them. The school provided that Andy would be on leave through Christmas vacation, thanks to the backup of her long-time colleagues and friends of the kindergarten program. From many sources — intuitions, trying to see through the professional masks of doctors we were consulting, and weighing the significance of my out-of-body vision — Andy and I were beginning to understand that I would not be going back to teaching children. My vocation and calling of the past thirty years was over. What the future held was hidden.

The Open Boat

The council of teachers had scheduled a meeting with the parents to speak with them about sharing responsibility for carrying the class. Many were hoping this would be on an interim basis while sorting through the implications of my critical illness. I was concerned that the parents would not know what to say to their children in this stormy passage. How could they? So I penned the following letter to be read at the parent meeting:

> December 10, 2005
> Dear Fourth Grade Parents,
>
> I am sorry I cannot be with you for this momentous meeting. Instead, I have written you a letter and asked Cecelia, who has a particularly strong connection with this class, to read it to you. First some musings, then practical matters.
>
> Thank you and your children for all your compassion and affection. Your strong good will flows toward me like a child's prayer, "...no fear can come near, but only love for all around me here." You and many friends continue to weave a garment of protection for me much like the robe

of light that St. Martin was wrapped in for the kindness of sharing his own cloak with a beggar.

I have mentioned before that I feel like I am reborn. It is a paradox to taste the sweetness of life more intensely while seriously ill. Another paradox is that I feel younger, more balanced and lucid than I have felt in years. My sense of humor is undiminished. I think of our great delight when a child is born. At such times we see the world, each other, and the new baby with open hearted reverence and renewed joy. Suddenly, I am waking up in a new way to Andy, Claire, Rosie, the children, you, my colleagues, friends, and innocent passersby. This receptive recognition is the way life is in its essence when the mundane makes way for the miraculous.

Ultimately, what is most important to us is our family, our children. The children are our mirrors and teachers as we are their guardians and guides. We invest our hope in them and offer our support. Our aspiration is that they may reach beyond where we left off and fully realize and fulfill their potential, their humanity. We are all on a path of self-discovery, ever casting off the old and growing into the new. The ancient words "Die and Become" hint at this continuous process of self-transformation and renewal. Nature pictures this vividly for us in the birth of the butterfly (*psyche*) emerging from its sleep in a jeweled coffin. Miraculously, hidden from sight in the dark cocoon, the caterpillar that spun its own shroud emerges, transformed into a butterfly! The children all saw this wondrous rebirth in first grade when Natalie brought in a cocoon. (I prayed it would hatch. They had no doubt.) We were patient, expectant. We released the monarch into the bright blue sky one autumn day.

Through the lens of my illness, the question of balance in life is seen in high relief. Balance is at the heart of our humanity and health. Balance is also crucial to the form of education we offer. The uprightness and balance won in early childhood is a lifelong gift. This gift of self-propulsion delights my grandson Otto (and his doting grandparents).

A tremendous power of will to stand upright and explore the world impels this achievement. How significant it is that our feet are planted on the ground and our hands are free to create and work. Your children, in ways unique to each, strongly carry will power. How we foster at home and school *education of the will* is crucial to their fulfilling their potential. More strongly than ever before, I experience the abundant will forces in this remarkable constellation of children, strengthening one another in mysterious ways. I am filled with confidence in the progressive unfolding of their capacities in relationship to each other and in proportion to their active interest in the world.

But the earth is shaking beneath our feet. Through the shadow of my illness, we walk toward an unknown future.

I have been given a gift of seeing our children and the extended family of our community with new eyes. It is a most beautiful sight. I am standing in the doorway between the known past and the unknown future. Without knowing the details, we still know deep down that *it is the nature of my illness that I will not be able to continue as the teacher of these wonderful children.* Let that thought ring in silence for a moment....

As the form of my illness becomes better known to you, as it is becoming known to Andy and me, you will understand why I cannot continue doing what I have done for nearly thirty years.

You have heard only a little about my surgery for brain cancer and are wondering what comes next. My realization that I will not continue with teaching is both quite objective and tremendously moving at the same time. This assessment is based on what I have learned thus far in the midst of many unknowns. Andy and I will drive to the Dana-Farber Cancer Institute in Boston on Tuesday, December 13, to learn the details of a comprehensive treatment that includes allopathic and complementary medicine. Our dear friends, doctors Stewart and Brigitte Kaufman, arranged this visit. Several powerful therapies for the healing process have already begun. We will also receive a second opinion on optimal treatment and an overview of the illness from the oncologist at Albany Medical Center. We are in consultation and have begun a therapeutic process already with Dr. Hertle. So the Wards are in high gear. We are researching, consulting with experienced professionals, and seeking out new friends who have weathered similar life-changing challenges.

Andy, my daughters, and your prayerful attention are absolute anchors for me. The few visitors I have had are very encouraged and encouraging when they sense my equilibrium in circumstances that are in all honesty "life threatening." But real life cannot be threatened. Life is self-sustaining and flows through us continuously. We have no say over the hour of our departure.

In Norse mythology, the Norns (the Fates) determine the hour of birth and the hour of death beside the fountain where the water of life continually flows. I could be wrong, but my intuition tells me that I have an inner, artistic work to do, much different from my active outer role in the school. I am as elated at this prospect as I am saddened at the thought of no longer serving as an amused grandfather among your lively offspring. Such is life.

My therapeutic regimen, as far as we can foresee, will likely require about thirty radiation treatments for this particular form of brain cancer. This will take six and a half weeks. The allopathic radiation treatment is dramatically enhanced by complementary therapies employed to strengthen the immune system. Among these is a carefully regulated treatment of Iscador administered intravenously one time per week and subcutaneously three times per week. This mistletoe extract, developed by Rudolf Steiner and Dr. Ita Wegman, is widely known in Europe for treating various types of cancer. A month's convalescence in Switzerland, two weeks at the Lucas Clinic in Arlesheim and two weeks at the Casa di Cura in Ascona is likely. I am eager to take on this challenge in the climate of prayerful support that surrounds me.

It is self-evident, once one has enough information, that I can no longer be a class teacher. I am at least as surprised by this as you are. In fact, I am astounded! But my path has taken a dramatic turn that affects us all. You as the parents of the class and the council of teachers responsible for the health of the class will join forces to build the circle of support around the children that will sustain them and their new teacher through this transition. Your devotion to their well being and their own healthy resilience will see them through. I, far but near, am woven into this supportive fabric. I have great faith that the right teacher will come to rally the children with your blessing and the council's whole-hearted support. This may not be the story we all had in mind, but "Life is what happens when you're busy making plans."

You now need to "sleep on all this." There is a lot to come to terms with before one finds peace and embraces what is new and unknown.

If you are standing in the doorway with me looking in two directions, toward the landscape of the past and the mysterious new world of the future, you might feel as I do—somehow our children already know. After all, they are the Children of the Future.

As you take in what you have heard this evening, meditate especially on how you will bring this to your child in the most positive and trusting light. I will do the same. Perhaps a story, a letter, or a poem will arise that will be helpful. Meanwhile, I know I live in their hearts and your hearts as you live in mine. To life!

Your friend,
William

       Ω

That invitation for a poem worked overnight. It wrote itself the next day and put our situation in picture form. It was read to the class and sent home to the parents:

THE OPEN BOAT

The whole tribe from the oldest grandmother to the youngest babe in arms sat in circle at the edge of the sea. A fire burned in their midst as the eldest among them stood to speak.

> "Stand up my brave young crew.
> I have a gift to give to you.
> I bring it from the farther shore.
> I have been there and back.
> Now I will sail no more.
> You are young and I am old.
> For you, many journeys lie ahead.
> Expect storm-tossed seas and hidden reefs.
> Count on safe harbors and the mercy of strangers.
> From this day on I stay on solid ground.
> The lighthouse fire I will tend,
> Safe harbor for your journey's end."

There was silence in the circle as they drank in his words. Had he said he would no longer be their captain? The fire crackled, and he continued his story.

> "You have all you need for now,
> All that I can give.
> Stay awake, find your balance,
> Learn, grow, and live.
> Each of you must shape your own oar,
> Use the wood of Yggdrasil.
> Carve it straight and strong to fit your hand
> And wake your sleeping will.
> Together craft a sturdy ship
> To ride the pounding waves.
> Carve a dragon for its bow.
> Fear not and be brave.
> Raise high the straightest mast of pine,

Weave a sail to catch the wind
To bear you through the storm
Against the driving rain.
Forge shields of thick bull's hide
To protect you from all harm.
Keep your eye on Polaris,
Your faithful guide all night.
Learn the stars' sacred lore,
To steer by their light.
Aim toward the rising sun
Born from the surging sea.
Spirit wind billow your sails to eternity."

*Silence filled the circle, but for the crackling of
    the fire.
The captain threw on another log.
The flames flickered higher.*

"Answer this riddle if you ken.
  Where does firelight come from?"
"From the wood of trees."
"Where does wood come from?"
"The great tree that unites
  heaven, earth and sun."
"Where does the fire go when it is set free?'
"It sheds its light into the night, warming you
    and me."
"What remains when the fire goes out?"
"Only ash remains."
"What springs forth from dark ash?"
"New trees rise again."
"What lifts their mighty trunks and spreads
    their branches wide?"
"The sun's loving light that fills all hearts with
    life."

"You have answered well.
  Soon I will give the gift.

But not before we give our thanks
For light and life and health.
Pass the sacred bowl to make our circle whole.
Let the Mead of Inspiration
Be the fountain in your soul."

They passed the bowl from hand to hand,
Each one took a sip.
It was fire in the belly
And honey on the lip.

"Wave tossed, I was lost, alone,
And could not find my way.
In fear and dread I wondered
'Would the sea be my grave?'
Then the lightning flashed!
And the sun broke through the rain.
The rainbow bridge arched 'cross the sky
And down to earth again.

I set my feet upon blood red,
Climbed higher through orange fire,
Was embraced by sun's yellow gold
And heard the heavenly choir.
There my brother, guide, and friend
Whispered words to me
And touched my body's earthly clay
To set my spirit free.

Then I fell back to earth below
And in my boat I woke.
The sea was calm, the storm was past.
Gulls circled, soared, and laughed.

Now—
Here in my heart,
Burns a sacred flame.
Nothing can ever put it out

For I know who I am.
And I know you
Live in me,
As I live in you,
A circle whole of many parts,
In the sunlight of the heart.

— — —

So my small boat drifted
Over the sea of blue,
As I gazed up to heaven,
With nothing more to do.
I am borne on the sea's broad back.
My guide holds the tiller.
We sail the pulsing tide
Of the sea that rolls forever.

One token I bring back,
This small and simple gift
That in a time of doubt
Will your spirit lift.
Take this little candle-boat
With light's tender love,
Lit from the living sun,
Overflowing from above,
May you find in its gentle flame,
Your soul's purpose,
Your spirit's aim."

With deepest respect for all the gifts you bring to share with
your brothers and sisters,
            Love,
            William Ward, Advent 2005

(A gnome-made Viking ship candle boat, thanks to the selfless assistance of my close friend Leif, was delivered to each
child at Christmas.)

CAPTAIN BUZZ BUZZ

DESPITE MY CONVICTION THAT I still had earthly work to do guided by instructions from the spiritual world, in "fact" the odds were five to one against me for survival beyond a year. And there was a serious/comical problem in addition to the cancer. I was manic with the pristine joy of new life. Sleep was impossible. I had to pretend to sleep to keep everyone's anxiety level down. Rest and quiet were crucial for my recovery from surgery. Unfortunately, these longed-for healing qualities were diametrically opposed by my anti-inflammatory medication, DECADRON.

It's a universal experience that when the alarm sounds, one gets the familiar jolt of adrenalin prescribed by millennia of evolutionary development. The saber tooth tiger is extinct, but phones are everywhere. (Even Alexander Graham Bell stuffed his phone with cloth so it would not interrupt his meditations.) I am not an endocrinologist, but like any cogitating mammal I can observe my internal responses to sudden stimuli, especially around the heart. I'd compare Decadron to an unflinching squeeze of the adrenal glands. Mercifully, not everyone has as strong a reaction as I had; the kind of post-operative psychosis I experienced is relatively rare. Dr. German's goal was to wean me as quickly as possible. The dosage was immediately halved to eight milligrams, then four, then two, then one, then one-half, all in a span of two weeks. The tapering off was necessary to ensure a smooth landing rather than a crash. Meantime, I had become a speed freak. I did not sleep for two and a half weeks.

My sleep substitute was the "deadman" posture of yoga. Dutifully I would "take my afternoon nap" and retire at a reasonable hour at night. As I lay in bed without stirring, I felt a peace and relaxation such as I had never known before. I felt the *prana,* the breath of life, coursing throughout my body. My circulatory and rhythmic systems were in a dance of revitalization, streaming vivifying blood to every living cell. The infinitely ramifying nerves were filled with the light of breath. Twining serpents rising to the winged sun of the caduceus staff was a radiant picture of my inner processes. I had supposed this symbol of the medical profession was arcane wisdom, the meaning of which had desiccated to selling pharmaceuticals. But the experience of the rhythmic flow of my breath was inscribed by intertwined serpents along the axis of my spine, the core of bodily wisdom, until the winged sun overflowed with healing energy in heart and mind. The mysterious phrase from the Bible that had puzzled me for three decades, ever since a conversation with my friend John Gardner, became self-evident. "If thine eye be single, it will illuminate the whole body." My eye and I had become single. I had loosed my grip, the grip holding myself in perpetual teaching posture with all its agendas, plans, and responsibilities. I blissfully let go of maintaining my body in the grip of tension, as though consciousness had to take responsibility for the whole works. Now I was on the receiving end, being bathed in light, since giving over my body, soul, and spirit to the forces of rejuvenation.

I was floating on a sunlight river of grace.

Side effects of Decadron or divine mercy? Who cares? Let's not split hairs. It is not for nothing that people put "Breathe" on their bumper stickers. We have forgotten how. Now I remember.

I felt I understood how Rudolf Steiner and other great emissaries from spirit realms were so productive on so little sleep. Immersion in the stream of the breath is receiving "the breath of life," *prana, ruach, pneuma,* down to the toes. Chuang Tze says, "The wise man breathes through his heels." Try it and see.

But this was not sleep. Dreaming sleep, sound sleep, and deep sleep take one progressively deeper into spiritual realms. As we learn from Rudolf Steiner's spiritual scientific research, the "I" and *astral body* leave behind the *physical body* and *etheric body* for their nightly journey to heavenly realms. Etheric forces restore the wasted body to wholesome balance in sleep, when consciousness cannot interfere. The Garden blooms again. You do not need to be a student of spiritual science, or Anthroposophy, to be intrigued by the question, "What happens to 'me' when I go to sleep?" Sleep research makes me nod off. No colorful electrode-relayed EEG displays for me. The equipment does not reach that far into the cosmos.

If the Garden does not get restored at night, thanks to nervousness, haunting echoes of the day's anxieties, and the media parade of tragedies, crises, and fears, one greets the new day with diminished ego strength, reduced energy for life, and exposed nerves. The rat race begins again. You don't ever see cows race. They ruminate and dream. We are too caught up in the nerve-sense systems: over-stimulated, hyper, speedy.

Enter Captain Buzz Buzz. I had always respected sleep's deep importance. But now, like clockwork, through the mystery of circadian rhythms, Captain Buzz Buzz, my alter ego, would rise at the stroke of midnight, on the dot. Things to do, places to go! Sleep was for others. My refreshment felt complete. I could not continue to lie in bed. Consciousness was too beautiful to miss a moment. Let us be up and doing. With the caution of a cat burglar, I would creep out of my cozy bed and inch down the hall, avoiding certain floorboards. Once downstairs I could write in my journal, before insights precious to me vaporized. I felt that my life had expanded to mythological proportions and I needed to record anything vibrating with significance from the day.

It hurts my pride to attribute more than its due to Decadron. But without it, I certainly would not have been getting up in the night so soon after surgery. I had tried to stay within the peace of breathing but.... I was swamped with the beauty of soul experiences. It would be irreverent to say "my" soul experiences. I was just open to the grace continuously available but generally unknown to day consciousness. My high-fidelity, wi-fi, cellular, satellite-boosted receivers were tuned to all channels. News from the universe was being piped in and the volume was cranked.

I was tuned heart and mind to episodes from my life, dear friends (living and dead), music beyond beautiful, and a Technicolor eurythmy production of the New World Symphony with high-definition accuracy. Oh, yes, the Isis-Osiris myth recurred not before me, but in me—let's say in the theater of my mind.

Why sleep? Silent tears would stream from my eyes. I was out of myself, ecstatic. Call me delusional, "tripping," "touched by prophetic vision," "psycho," inspired—whatever. However one wants to categorize such waves of "feeling cognition," my nighttime consciousness was expansive. Anywhere I tuned my attention, that realm of experience—childhood, mythology, nature, music—would come on-line saturated with meanings. All was inscribed on my soul, be it cellular memory or *akashic* record. On my cerebral iPod, I can hear and see anything I want, or don't want. It's all there. But you have to be "out there" to hear it. And I was "out there."

One of the reasons for getting up in the night, aside from drying out my pillow from tears of joy, was getting a grip on myself. I was not haunted by fear of death or worries about the "progress of my illness." That I had given over to the Lord in irrevocable trust. The only way I could approximate "normal" was to write in the dead of night. Ah, the relief of linear consciousness, left to right, sequential rather than simultaneous. That was tough because my thoughts kept branching like neurons. When a synapse fired with an interesting digression, I would try to note it for subsequent follow up. Ha! There is a Sisyphean ordeal. There were fragments and shards of interesting things to be followed through later scattered on scraps, Post-its, legal pads, and my oak-embossed leather journal. Nonetheless, I soldiered on first with pen and paper. When I soon ran out of ink from my midnight musings, I realized, despite the soothing rhythmic activity of writing, I needed to switch to the keyboard. This was my only hope of storing hints quickly enough to meet the torrent of meaning coming my way. For the moment it was sufficient that the process of writing was helping me come back to myself.

After an hour and a half, I would steal back to bed, returning to the breath of life. Exactly an hour and a half later, Captain Buzz Buzz would step off the magic carpet ride of the breath, surreptitiously tiptoe out, and begin to write again. My rhythm was: 10:00 to midnight, "deadman" pose deep relaxation; midnight to 1:30, journaling; 1:30 to 3:00 a.m., "body of light" ongoing baptism; 3:00 to 4:30, journaling; 4:30 a.m. to 6:30, so-called sleep.

"How did you do last night?" asks Andy.

"Pretty well under the circumstances. I got up a couple of times, I had a really wonderful rest."

"But you need actual sleep."

"Hey, I'm trying over here, but someone is playing the New World Symphony, and they are piping it all over the neighborhood."

"Let's see if we can get your medication reduced more quickly. You've got to sleep."

The condition persisted for two and a half weeks. One of the beneficial side effects of the Decadron was that I could tend to business at night with an attention to detail worthy of a tax accountant. In addition to philosophical ramblings and personal dialogues with dear ones, Captain Buzz Buzz became Memo King. There were things I needed taken care of for my recovery and only I knew what verbiage to crank out to do the job: public communiqués, poems for the class, memos for administration and the development office, insurance questions, questions for my doctors, beginning an ad hoc filing system for the blizzard of notes wishing me well. There was no time in the day. That was reserved for family and peace and one hour for a visitor. I tried not to talk too much like a mad rapper. Instead I attempted to portray a peaceful grandfather, to the extent my busy mind allowed.

Flashing in neon on my agenda were the Children of the Future. I felt myself a messenger. I also felt that my illness was part of a much larger story that had to do with them and why I am writing this book. I needed to touch base with a few people who would listen in an open-hearted way to what I could only lamely articulate about the Children of the Future.

I felt like a college student writing a term paper against a deadline. My computer was smoking. Here is an example of midnight-oil labor, as I prepared questions for a post-operation consultation with Dr. German. We still didn't have any real information.

QUESTIONS FOR DOCTOR GERMAN

Tuesday, 11/28/06

Thank you Dr. German, I am so grateful for your intervention.

1. How many chemo treatments?
2. What is the time frame for this meeting?
3. What is the spectrum of possible reactions to the medication? No doubt it varies from individual to individual. Not having had powerful drugs in my body for years, my reactions to certain medications have been extreme.
4. Lifting, physical activity, what's allowed when?
5. What alternative therapies to chemo would you suggest we explore?
6. What is a typical reaction to chemotherapy, or is it so correlated with the subtleties of the body's chemistry as to be individualized?
7. In your opinion is there a relationship between the physical manifestation of the illness and the whole psychological matrix out of which the tumor grew? What, in your view, is the relationship of the chemotherapy, which I assume is operating on primarily a bodily physical-chemical basis and the more inward soul qualities in the healing process?
8. Statistically, what are we talking about here in mortality/ longevity for this type of tumor? Is there data for patients who include so-called alternative treatments? Is there any research on this available in layman's terms?
9. When should treatment begin if we choose that direction?
10. I assume we can opt out at any time.
11. Please characterize the side effects.

12. Over longer periods of time what rhythmic monitoring is advisable to ensure the illness process is held in check and does not recur?

13. How many therapeutic cycles of chemo might be called for over five years, over ten years, fifteen, or twenty?

14. The brain is separate from the body, isn't it, bathed in cerebral spinal fluid? What is your mental model of how the chemical substances release their effectiveness through the targeted area?

15. Am I right in thinking that the rest of the resilient body endures a chemical assault on behalf of "neutralizing" the focal point of the illness? The body's regenerative powers are great. The weekly swings between chemical assault and recovery sound challenging. Is there a more moderate approach possible or is it best to hit it hard to ensure it does not recur?

16. What is your understanding of the rate of recurrence for my age group: fifty-nine-year-old, male, with healthy life habits?

17. Are there statistics available on what demographic groups choose chemo vs. alternative therapies and statistically compiled success rates that you could refer us to?

18. If I were your father, what would you recommend for me?

No sooner finishing one memo, I would start another. Let's not digress to the thirty-eight–point memo I wrote to my friends in administration and development. They probably shook their heads in consternation, saying, "I thought he was supposed to be resting? Sedate him. Let go already!" But for me, "letting go" meant identifying loose ends and passing the baton responsibly. Instead of clinging to responsibilities, I was trying to shuck them as fast as possible, though a four-page memo might not look like it.

So I am thankful to have made the acquaintance of Captain Buzz Buzz for his management skills. I cannot fathom or accept an educational system that has more than five million kids on Ritalin. Does that have anything to do with the mission of the Children of the Future? But for me on my midnight ramblings, I must say Decadron knows how to get stuff done. Besides, it was prescribed by my doctor. He ought to know.

ISCADOR

IN THE WEEK BEFORE my surgery, Dr. Margaretha Hertle had recommended and initiated two therapies to work with my illness. These treatments she prescribed were complementary to the allo-pathic regimen of radiation and chemotherapy that would begin after my recovery from surgery. The first of these complementary cancer treatments comprised infusions and injections of Iscador. So, while Captain Buzz Buzz sped around by night, my beloved Iscador had exactly the opposite effect. Under the influence of infusions of this mistletoe extract, time would slow down to an absolute standstill—time to see the daylight silently streaming in to caress the far wall. How beautiful were the flowing designs of wood grain on doors and cabinets, suggestive of sunsets and still waters. Why read when I can see? Ripples of thought subside and my mind becomes a still mirror, a reflecting being—content-less contentment floating on the river of life. MELLLLOOOOOW-NESS. Here was the "Peace that passeth all understanding." Cancer, Schmancer, Romancer. What was this miraculous substance, Iscador? Who had ever heard of it?

This much I knew: Thirty-three doses of radiation focused on the brain-tumor site have a powerful effect on the whole body. Does the concept "sledge hammer" ring a bell? My liver was working overtime. Anything that makes your hair fall out is not exactly an elixir of health. Necessary, yes. Destructive by design, yes. Radiation is tolerable, but the immune system takes a beating and is compromised. It's a choose-your-poison situation, using the focused death ray to preserve life. Therefore, anyone facing cancer, or serious illness of any kind, is eager to learn of whatever can boost the immune system. Why? Because the immune system produces killer cells (our friends) that seek and destroy cancer cells that have run amok. They kill without mercy, which is a good thing. The cancer cells failed to sign the non-proliferation treaty. Their greedy and ultimately self-destructive agenda must be stopped. These renegades ("We don't care nothing for your stinkin' badges....") can reproduce at alarming, geometric rates. They must be nipped in the bud. They damage the healthy functioning of tissues and organs that are properly integrated into the balance of the whole body. A robust immune system detects the culprits. Macrophages ("great eaters") and leukocytes (white blood cells), among other warriors on the front lines of the body's defenses, eat the upstarts. When the rogues invade, production of killer cells in the bone marrow increases. Blood tests can monitor, among the many constituents of blood, these macrophages and white blood cells mobilized to combat illness. But, if already compromised, the immune system can also be overwhelmed by illness.

The manifestation of cancer is a late stage of physical processes a long time in the making. From a holistic perspective, the confluence of factors that contribute to the triggering of cancer include environmental carcinogens in the air and in the food chain; genetic predisposition; habits of mind such as joylessness, fear, compulsive criticality, and anxiety; regulatory disorders on a cellular level from stress, improper diet, lack of sleep; vocational stress; lack of warmth in childhood; biographical factors and soul wounds; poor self-esteem; and social factors like alienation and loneliness. Why not throw in *chi* blockage and bad *karma?*

How did this spectrum of negativity make me feel? Under siege? Depressed? At the bottom of a monkey pile? No, I felt intrigued, interested, activated, and challenged to know myself. Apparently I had been living with a stranger: me—my unrecognized self. The cancer was like a red rooster crowing "Rise and Shine." The wake up call for me was to make systemic changes of deep-seated habits that would let the river of life flow freely again. To do this I needed grace, courage, and inner activity.

Cancer is highly individualized. The patient could draft from self-observation a chart of surmised factors. This intellectual approach—apportioning percentages to hypothetical causes and factoring in the Shadow with its contributions of doubt, fear, inadequacy, guilt, and bad attitude could light up fruitful therapeutic paths or have a net effect of precisely zero. It all depends on imponderable virtues that cannot be weighed or measured: Honesty toward oneself, openness, receptivity, generosity, listening, patience, flexibility, reverence, courage, compassion, attentiveness, faith, love, levity, joy, willingness, positivity, equanimity, forgiveness. These are the wellsprings that make all of us fully human and alive. Incorporating these virtues—now that would be a boost to the immune system! This is soul work I want to do for my own healing, regardless of the "progress" of the disease. Whatever inner turning I can effect in my soul in thinking, feeling, and willing decreases the likelihood of resurgence of my illness. This is not a plea bargain, not "Give me another chance, Judge, and I promise to go straight." This is, "Thank you, wise spiritual guidance; thank you, bodily wisdom; thank you, Teacher-Cancer for this grace to work on myself."

Who said, "We are all headed toward death. Some people just don't know it"? Walls of DENIAL erected to defend oneself from fears of abandonment, annihilation, extinction, and the cold void can dissolve at the touch of a healing hand. In this sense, cancer is our collaborator in breaking down such walls. There are two poles of possibility: "I am in a fight for my life against cancer, my mortal enemy. Die, you bastard!" Or, "Cancer, teach me what I need to learn to change my life. I resolve to work with you to discover and transform my Self." There is a huge divide between these imaginations of the being of cancer. Summon both for the battle.

For now, my cells are happy. Iscador, you are my true friend. Sunlight is flowing like honey through my veins and into my heart. Let it flow. It's time to rest my eyes and just be....

These hour-long Iscador infusions, prescribed by my primary-care physician, who has researched and experienced its efficacy through her medical practice, were followed by blissful naps. My temperature prior to the infusion and after my rest were carefully monitored and noted. Cancer patients, especially those recovering from radiation and chemo, are sensitive to cold. Why not? Their life forces have taken a beating. My "normal" temperature since treatment has been in the vicinity of 97.4 degrees. A slight rise in temperature, often less than a degree, after the infusion was a good sign. Cancer is a "cold" illness. It is the opposite of an inflammatory illness. A little inflammation in the case of cancer is regarded as a good thing. Have you noticed that you get as many variations in temperature readings as the number of thermometers used regardless of which orifices are being measured? I have heard that 98.6 degrees, once considered the normal human temperature, has altered over time. "Normal" is nearly a degree lower than it once was. Interesting.... Turn the air-conditioning down. We are wasting heat. What is this tendency toward coldness, coldness in all respects?

After once-per-week infusions, each one a six-hour mini-vacation, for seven weeks, the protocol changed. From then on, my twenty-milliliter ampule of Iscador was subcutaneously injected three times weekly into my spare tire. I proudly overcame my aversion to needles. The needles were so fine that an injection felt halfway between a mosquito bite and a weak bee sting. After my morning injection, I was to rest for at least half an hour as the Iscador entered the blood stream to the cheers of enthusiastic macrophages. A slight pink spot on the skin was the only sign that reinforcements were on the way.

I knew Iscador was my friend, but a friend about whom I knew nothing. A little research was in order. From *Grieve's Herbal:*

History — Mistletoe was held in great reverence by the Druids. They went forth clad in white robes to search for the sacred plant, and when it was discovered, one of the Druids ascended the tree and gathered it with great ceremony, separating it from the oak with a golden knife. The mistletoe was always cut at a particular age of the moon, at the beginning of the year, and it was only sought for when the Druids declared they had visions directing them to seek it. When a great length of time elapsed without this happening, or if the mistletoe chanced to fall to the ground, it was considered as an omen that some misfortune would befall the nation. The Druids held that the mistletoe protected its possessor from all evil, and that the oaks on which it was seen growing were to be respected because of the wonderful cures which the priests were able to effect with it. They sent round their attendant youth with branches of the Mistletoe to announce the entrance of the new year. It is probable that the custom of including it in the decoration of our homes at Christmas, giving it a special place of honor, is a survival of this old custom. The curious basket of garland with which "Jack-in-the-Green" is even now occasionally invested on Mayday is said to be a relic of a similar garb assumed by the Druids for the ceremony of the mistletoe. When they had found it they danced round the oak to the tune of "Hey Derry down, down, down Derry!" which literally signified, "In a circle move we round the oak." Some oak woods in Herefordshire are still called *"the Derry";* and the following line from Ovid refers to the Druids' songs beneath the oak:

—Ad viscum Druidce cantare solebant—

Shakespeare calls it "the baleful Mistletoe," an allusion to the Scandinavian legend that Baldur, the god of Peace, was slain with an arrow made of mistletoe. He was restored to life at the request of the other gods and goddesses, and mistletoe was afterward given into the keeping of the goddess of Love, and it was ordained that everyone who passed under it should receive a kiss, to show that the branch had become an emblem of love, and not of hate.

(from an article in Wikipedia; en.wikipedia.org/)

Rudolf Steiner first suggested the use of mistletoe extract injections for the treatment of cancer as early as 1917, based on his spiritual scientific research. Ita Wegman, founder of the Lucas Clinic in Arlesheim, Switzerland, put his suggestions into practice. He also designed a machine for mistletoe extraction and gave indications for harvesting the mistletoe in spring and autumn for maximum potency of the anti-cancer cell toxins. Little did I know that the wheels were already turning that would lead me to the Lucas Clinic. The Gift of my illness would take me there on the wings of generosity. A benefactor had said to me, "Seek the treatment you need." So I did.

This is what I discovered. Since Steiner's time clinical research and experience surrounding the use of Iscador has intensified and spread. Quoting from the frontispiece of the book *Iscador: Mistletoe and Cancer Therapy,* here are some salient Iscador facts in a nutshell:

> Iscador is a prescription medicine in injectable form, developed in Europe.
> It has been in continuous use since 1917.
> It is the cancer drug most recognized by name in Germany.
> Over sixty percent of cancer patients in Germany use some form of mistletoe.
> Iscador is more often prescribed by oncologists and conventional physicians than by complementary physicians.
> Millions of doses of Iscador are sold worldwide each year.
> Iscador is a Class-P homeopathic tincture of *viscum album* diluted to a clinically safe dosage.
> Over one hundred studies have been done on Iscador.
> Let the word go forth about Iscador. "Seek and ye shall find."

Mistletoe therapy has been used in Germany and Switzerland for cancer treatment for over eighty years. It takes a while for us to hear about these things. Remember how recently the Food and Drug Administration prohibited importing drugs from Canada because they might not be safe? This strikes me as a similar situation. If you happened to be plugged into the media (a vice I do not indulge), you will be saturated with advertisements for

Ambien, Lunesta, vitamins, Lipitor, heart medications, Viagra, Cyalis, and various products to keep you from getting headaches, high blood pressure, and indigestion from watching the news. But you will never see or hear a word about Iscador. Oh, well.... I wonder when health insurance will hear about Iscador? It seems my insurance plan, with a $6,000 deductible for catastrophic illness, allows any number of MRIs at $2,000 to $3,000 a pop, but not one dime for Iscador. I confess to being slightly afraid of mentioning it to my oncologist. I don't want to undermine our working relationship by bringing up something that has not been "proven," whatever that means according to the scientific orthodoxy that currently holds sway. I'm more of an "if it's good enough for the Druids, it's good enough for me" kind of guy. If Rudolf Steiner's spiritual scientific research points to mistletoe, I am ready to receive its benefits. On the theme of proof: "By their fruits ye shall know them." It took only about forty years to "prove" that smoking is bad for your health, though it was blatantly obvious to all from the beginning. Time is short. I don't have the patience to wait for the folks in white coats, with their genetically engineered lab rats, to figure out whether they can allow this plant extract to be used by the public. Instead, I'm going to rely on the Swiss, who live in a land that keeps its nose out of wars, is the safe repository of the gold of the world, and is a premier distributor of top-grade chocolate. Now I am going to make a bold statement. If I had to choose between chocolate and Iscador, I'd choose Iscador every time. Fortunately, I don't have to make that choice.

The mistletoe plant itself is beautiful and mysterious. It is a *saprophyte* that lives by the hospitality of the host tree. It never touches the ground. A sticky seed, excreted by a bird, adheres to a branch. The mistletoe seed penetrates the branch bark of its host tree only as far as the life-giving cambium layer. The wood of the tree forms a protective wall around the base of the mistletoe plant, which continues its slow growth toward the periphery. It may take three years to produce the first pair of oblong-round leaves. The simple leaves, reminiscent of the simple seed leaves of flowering plants, have the gesture of two hands open in a chalice to the sun.

By the third year the stem begins to branch, each branch producing only a pair of leaves per year, forming a spherical community by the seventh year. The mature female plant unfolds an undifferentiated green cylindrical flower in May, which ripens into an egg-like form that becomes a white, translucent, shining berry by the time of the Winter solstice.

Birds love it.

If a wise philanthropist should happen to read this book, please remember what I am about to say. I have a message for you. This is a pearl of great price. A good deed would be to fund further research and development of Iscador to document its healing properties on this North American continent. Iscador is a gift. Perhaps it is a sacrament. May the healing might of this remedy benefit all who seek it. May its healing power become a balm for the Children of the Future.

From my current perspective, it's remarkably farsighted that I had written a play for fourth graders twenty-six years ago, in which mistletoe had a prominent role. In the fourth grade, coinciding with the end of the golden years of childhood, the Waldorf school language arts curriculum features Norse mythology. Now, twenty-six years later, I reread what I once wrote, searching for prophetic clues about mistletoe and pondering the mysterious circling of my own karma. The Norse gods open the play with homage to the sun god:

> **Aesir:** Radiant Baldur, gold son of Odin,
> Thy beautiful brow beams bright over heaven,
> Best loved of gods, bearer of light,
> Yet death's dreary dreams darken your night.
>
> – – –
>
> **Baldur:** A dark dream of death
> Overshadows my bed,
> Foretelling my fall
> To the land of the dead.

Later in the play, Baldur's mother rallies the gods to action to save Baldur from death:

> **Frigga:** Without my son, no one will live,
> Let all the world a promise give,
> Let birds and beasts, stones and trees,
> Fire and fish, old age, disease,
> Wind and water, iron and ice,
> Vow they will not take his life,
> For by his life we all may live,
> So let the world this promise give.

(last to be asked to help save Baldur is the mistletoe)

> **Frigga:** Mistletoe, moonlit mistletoe,
> Twining up so high,
> You could not wish my son to die,
> You are so small, what harm could you do,
> Yet I must ask also of you,
> Do you vow Baldur never will die
> While shining Sol crosses the sky?

Before a response comes, Loki, disguised as a crone, intervenes, preventing mistletoe's promise. We won't make that mistake. When Frigga leaves, Loki climbs the tree and carves a deadly dart of mistletoe. With this poison dart, Loki, the trickster, engineers Baldur's death at the hand of his blind brother, Hodur. Baldur dies and descends to the House of the Dead. After Ragnarök, the Twilight of the Gods, Baldur resurrects in the newborn earth:

> **Aesir:** Sail the dark sea
> Beyond world's end
> Till all evil hearts
> By fire have been cleansed.
> Beyond Ragnarok
> When Yggdrasil burns,
> The dawn of new life
> Seeks your return...

(Baldur and Nanna appear behind the Aesir)

> Pour forth your love
> On the new-born earth,
> Light the new world
> With joyous rebirth!

That ancient story is also my story. Thor battles the world-encircling serpent just as I fight cancer. But after the battle comes the resurrection. Circle of cancer friends, may we all live to see that resurrection day! Thank you, Mistletoe.

CYPRESS BAPTISM

THE OTHER TREATMENT WAS a form of hydrotherapy called Oil Dispersion Baths. Now, a year later, as a cancer survivor, I am continuing these and other therapies, trying to understand how and why I have been spared and how in the mysterious world these substances are so efficacious.

Naked as a jaybird I descend into a large tub of warm, clear blue water. The temperature of the bath is calibrated to be one degree below my body temperature. The fragrance of cypress oil is in the air, and miniscule droplets of cypress suffuse the water. I relax. As I immerse myself, the tiny droplets adhere to the surface of my body. My heart "unwinds." The bath mistress, dear nurse Margaret, fans and swirls the water to wherever it is needed, feathering across the kidneys, liver, and heart, relieving little knots of tension in the muscles, encouraging flow along energy meridians of the body. Twenty minutes later, I emerge from the bath, squeegee off the slippery water, and, still wet, wrap myself in a cotton blanket. Then I lie down and am snugly swaddled in woolen blankets. Only my face is exposed to the air.

I am a mummy. For the next hour in my cocoon, I am bound in body, but my thoughts roam freely. No meetings, no appointments, no errands, no sensory stimulus, I have been slowed to a complete standstill. Now, at last, I am free to meet myself. Can the mind also gradually slow down until all the ripples of that sensitive medium subside toward clarity and stillness? Or will the ripple effects of continual mental/emotional exertion override this opportunity for self-reflection? Whatever the case, I ain't goin' nowhere. That in itself is a major breakthrough. For a timeless moment I am *this*. A Beatles song drifts through: "What do you see when you turn off the lights? / I can't tell you, but I know it's mine."

In the cocoon, the miraculous metamorphosis takes place. A caterpillar goes in, a butterfly emerges.

Cancer is a manifestation of imbalance on all levels, not just the physical level where it can belatedly be detected. We all harbor cancer cells, but the healthy functioning of the immune system discovers and eliminates them. What is the immune system? How do cancer cells get a foothold? Theories abound. Individual variables defy standardization. The interpenetrating, dynamic complexities of bodily processes confound linear thinking and schematic categorization. The insurgents have penetrated the perimeter and could be hiding anywhere. Homeland security is overwhelmed. The invading anarchists want to overthrow the existing regime. They refuse to take the oath of allegiance, "One body, indivisible...." In this situation, what can stimulate our highest powers of healing?

I don't pretend to know. What I thought I "knew" has been overturned by my illness. Like the snake handlers from Gnosos to Walapi in Hopi land, cancer, too, has much to teach in handling the deadly serpent. A healer, like Moses, holds the serpent power in his hands as pestilence comes wave on wave. This face of cancer is a great teacher. For one grappling with cancer, "What does cypress or any other plant out there have to do with me? Don't I have more urgent concerns for God's sake?"

Soon after Dr. Hertle's prescribed treatments began, I would learn that the allopathic paradigm was adamant about prescribing radiation therapy and Temodar chemotherapy for this virulent form of cancer. Bring on the radiation, bring on the chemo, I want to live! However, those are death forces. They are designed

Hold fast to the Great Mother —
Earth, Matrix, Mater,
Gaia, Natura, Madonna —
Warmed in your embrace,
We grow heavenward,
Lifted by sunlight's grace.

So ramifying roots
Delving into matter's night,
Let yearning limbs unfold
Into the fruits of light.

I, Cypress, am the axis,
Between the root and crown,
I am the mighty column
Binding heaven to the ground.
Feet planted in the soil,
I hold high heaven's dome.
I am the tree bridge
Between the stars and stones.
I feel the waves' pulse on the shore,
I hear bedrocks' deepest tones.
I inhale air's sweet breath,
And exhale the wild wind's moan.

I, Cypress,
Stand upright;
Frozen form of flame,
I offer up my essence
To those who know
My name.
I turn sunlight to scented wood
Till fire sets my spirit free
And gray ash
Alone remains
To receive the fallen seeds.

I harvest seas of light,

I embody health.
My sun-imbued elixir
Will fortify the Self.
Soil and air
Become my flesh,
I am the sacred tree
Rooted below,
Illumined above
For eternity.

Do you think I make these little ditties up, or is "someone" speaking out of the Being of Cypress? Mind you, I don't have a clue how one can extract an oil from a particular plant, whirl a couple of drops through a vortex into a tub, absorb it through the pores, and have it emerge into a powerful Imagination of the Being of Cypress who is willing to speak to this infirm vessel. All I can say is, "I want cypress on my side." Cypress can do things for me that I can't possibly do for myself, like transform sunlight to a healing oil.

For my condition, cypress was a crucial agent of transformation. The signature of my cancer was unformed proliferation of unwanted cellular growth. Where is the pruning swat team? The immune system is on siesta. For God's sake, Macrophages: mobilize! This is out of control. Poison ivy has crept in under the fence and is choking the garden. Enter cypress: flame shaped, force of form, uprightness, evergreen, straight grained, sunlight bearer, centered in itself, integrator of cosmic forces. Cypress embodies ego forces, forming forces, sculptural forces that my watery, acquiescing nature needs.

In conversations with Andy and Dr. Hertle, we realized that I had not provided enough protection for myself. I had generously given of myself too much to my students, to the school, to parents, and the school community without restraint. I had desired to please others without respect for my own needs. I had sacrificed to an unhealthy degree self-initiated creativity and soul space to institutional pressures. Also, I had internalized other people's difficulties or conflicts more than I realized, more than was healthy.

This one-sidedness was a suitable habitat
and proliferate. Egoity and its physiol⌐
immune system, had dropped their gu
dence of cancer, the integrity, virtues
cypress were called for. Clear boundaɪ⌐
a class teacher. Saying "No" was, for my dispos⌐
had to learn the hard way.

How does one explain the effects of cypress or other oils from ⌐
spiritual scientific point of view, the perspective of anthroposophically extended medicine? As context I will quote notes from a talk
by Dr. Thomas von Rottenburg who has worked therapeutically
and as a researcher with essential oils for the past sixteen years:

> Therapies in general have four potential "entrances" to our
> Being ...:
>
> Surgery, physical therapy and certain massage tech-
> niques, as well as allopathic drugs, have their main effect on
> the *physical* substance, the "earth" element [of the body].
>
> Acupuncture works directly into the life forces, or *etheric*
> sphere, related to the "water" element, which brings life to
> physical substance and can be perceived as the "uplifting"
> forces that allow a tree to grow up, or the apple to be formed
> out of the elements of earth....
>
> Most homeopathy and Bach flower remedies, as well as
> aromatherapy, address the level of the *astral body*, the bodily
> entity that allows human beings and animals to express feel-
> ings. It is related to our soul life, to our breathing and to
> the air element. There is a very close relation between our
> breathing life and our feelings. The ancients recognized the
> relation of the stars to our emotional life, hence the name
> "astral."
>
> The fourth level has to do with our *ego* ["I"] and ego
> organization, which is the level spoken to by the oil disper-
> sion baths....

Dr. von Rottenburg discusses the rejection by the immune
system of organ transplants: "We human beings are so much
individualized, we don't tolerate foreign organs." Then he speaks

of the connection between the immune system and the "I"
ization:

Our "search," our pain and our joy in life, is to find our individual path. Our unique individuality, our spiritual core, is
what we refer to as our ego. This has everything to do with
our immune system, which is closely tied to our warmth
organism [e.g., fever activates the immune system and is our
highest source of healing].

Later in the lecture: "When our individual ego forces are
exposed to the divine principle in an essential oil, that principle is
made available to our ego forces as a healing impulse.... The oil
dispersion process allows for a direct absorption...by the immune
system, the carrier of our ego forces."

The patient's will toward healing, his or her ego engagement
with the illness, is essential. For the therapy to be effective, the
individual must ask:

What is my soul forcing me to learn through this disease,
or what is meant by the disease?...In the end, all of our
illnesses are an expression of our inability to live up to
our own potential...we can see in our illnesses the "unre-
deemed" expression of our unused talents or potentials.

It's helpful to have a conceptual framework as context for
new ideas. But with the Grim Reaper breathing down my neck, I
needed no theoretical backup to justify my intense inner experiences with cypress and the series of oils prescribed since. As Emerson observed, "Spirit is that which is its own evidence."

Cypress has spoken to me.

ISIS AND OSIRIS

AFTER ONE OF MY cypress baths, I am lying in bed in the "dead man's pose." A temple maiden (actually my neighbor, Nicole) enters the darkened chamber to perform the ritual act of healing, the laying on of hands. She massages rhythmically my feet and calves with blackthorn oil. Every bone, joint, ligament, capillary, vein, artery, nerve, muscle, and whatever else is down there is receiving the reward of bodily existence. The head at the other end of this transaction, though wounded, has completely abdicated all responsibility of governance in favor of pure pleasure. Myriad cells are dancing in the streets and singing Hosannas of gratitude. Again, the body is filled with light and becomes light as a feather. What a gift of mercy.

As for evening's rest, Andy has abandoned the marital bed for the time being, knowing that Captain Buzz Buzz will begin his midnight rambles as the clock strikes twelve. The patient, awake but inert, enters the zone. Notes from my journal record the experience:

> It is a wonderful thing to have cypress tears. This holy water streams out of my eyes. Aromatic. How did this come to pass? The Therapeuta prepared the bath. Cypress, grand spirit, primal Being, you who knit together heaven and earth with the Tree of Life, deeply rooted, upright pillar — your form clarity be my own uprightness.
>
> Steps: immersion, chaotization, absorption of essence, swaddled sleep of bather, waking day consciousness, night awakening. Lying on my back, "sleeping," I am overcome by the realization that I am overflowing with cypress tears. I shake uncontrollably with gratitude and joy and incomprehension. I try to hold myself in, but I begin to quiver again and cover my face with my hands.

Be a man. Make sure you are not projecting. Cypress tears? Yes, cypress tears.

Then a stream of images flows through me. I know the story because I am a Waldorf teacher, but now I am not telling it. I am in it as it unfolds. Osiris, in his coffin, floats down the Nile and out to sea. I am in the coffin. Osiris, with his divine sister, Isis, has brought language, agriculture, peace, and harmony between heaven and earth to Egypt. Set, his destructive brother, devises a coffin. The one who fits exactly within receives this precious chest as a gift. Osiris fits perfectly. Set and his servants lock him in. Lead seals the seams. He is cast into the Nile and floats away, carried on the waters. Isis searches far and wide for him. He comes aground at Byblos and is absorbed into the body of a tree, a cypress tree. Osiris remains within this tomb until Isis can find and free him.

Isis's search brings her at last to Byblos. Birds and children tell her that the tree containing Osiris has been cut down and become the aromatic and upright central pillar of the temple. Isis becomes the nurse of the future king, a child, and awaits her beloved's release from the column. Ever helpful and knowing how to do magical things, Isis by night dips the royal infant by the heel into the flames of immortality. The king and queen catch her. The magic that would have made the child immortal is incomplete. As she reveals herself and tells her story, it becomes clear that Osiris is in the column. He is released. Isis and Osiris return to Egypt. Their reign is restored.

But the process of death and resurrection continues. This time, Set kills Osiris to rule in his stead. He has him dismembered and the pieces of the divine body are widely scattered to fourteen places. Isis gathers all the pieces of her brother-husband's body. Does one piece remain missing? (I need that missing piece.) When Osiris is reintegrated from his dismemberment, he becomes king of the afterlife.

There, in the afterlife, the judgment is given for each of us, O my brothers and sisters. Our heart is weighed against the feather of truth. We say our own name in the Hall of Judgment: I am Osiris William. The weighing tests the lightness of our heart against the feather of truth. If we are found worthy, we take our rightful place among the dead.

This is why I have cypress tears streaming out of my eyes. Osiris's and Isis's story is my story, your story. Take a bath of healing for your soul and body so the light of the spirit shines in your acts of the day. Then the temple will be rooted in earth and its central column will be illumined by the light of heaven.

I wrote that journal entry for my eyes alone. I unseal the journal here to hint at the soul's ferment in the presence of cancer. Writing in the journal in the middle of the night gave a space and time where I could begin to find some order in the simultaneity of my rapidly ramifying thoughts. I was, like the dismembered Osiris, trying to get myself back together again. Humpty Dumpty had a great fall and lay in pieces. Not to be grandiose, but struggling to find coherence in my experiences including the baths, I felt myself to be undergoing an *initiation*. The steps included "the temple sleep," "death," "dismemberment," "night journey," "encountering the shadow," "meeting the guardian," "forgiveness," "baptism-redemption," "resurrection," "rebirth," and "return."

I knew that the powerful pictures of my imagination as I lay in bed were "only" images, but they pointed to spiritual realities—the riddle of death and rebirth. I also found it emotionally overwhelming that the two drops of cypress, placed hours before in the bath, now streamed out my eyes with cypress fragrance in the middle of the night. The feeling of floating on the waters and being sustained by grace lifted me up. I identified so strongly with the images of my waking dream that I *participated* in the story of William/Osiris in the coffin and followed his transformation into a tree. It is mysterious that a story I had last reviewed eight years before for a main lesson was so deeply lodged in me that it could rise to the surface triggered by the healing effects of the baths.

Civilizations come and go. Isis and Osiris remain. Cypress remains. The archetypes, especially at times of chaos, fear, despair, and grave illness, abide with us as spiritual guides through the "valley of the shadow of death." These living imaginations point over the water to the farther shore—the spiritual world.

O My Angel

O my Angel, spread your wings
And bear me to the source of things—

Far into the world of light
Hidden in the heart of night.

O my Angel, let me sleep—
Bathe me in the star-bright deep.

Bathe my being bright and clean—
Heal me in the vast unseen.
—Arvia MacKaye Ege

Loony or Illumined

Gradually, I was becoming myself again. Hard to believe after the foregoing, but true. I was reintegrating, coming down to earth. But I was profoundly different inwardly. There was something I urgently wanted to communicate about the gifts of the Children of the Future. My illness opened me up to slough off my old skin, the dead habits and husks of outmoded thoughts. The living kernel of rebirth of consciousness was already sprouting. But I didn't have the words to frame the energy of the bursting, burgeoning seeds that I sensed in a new generation of children. I was too tongue-tied to speak about it and anxious that, by waiting too long, it would lose the energy of its revelation. It would seem ordinary or illusory.

The snide Inquisitor weasels into my doubts and opines: Obviously the author of these rantings is a lunatic supersaturated with self-serving "spiritual" projections unconsciously devised to save his own skin. The residual effects of drug-induced psychosis, coupled with a tenacious and totally unrealistic *joie d'vivre*, have made him zany and delusional. The swaddling he so prizes as part of his pseudo-scientific hydrotherapy is nothing more than infantile regressions and a misplaced desire to return to the womb. There is no scientific evidence that a so-called spiritual world exists — quite the contrary: the non-existence of evidence is evidence that there is no evidence for the existence of this hypothetical world. The much trumpeted first person pronoun "I" (which appears a little too often in this narrative to be above suspicion) has been determined by advanced imaging techniques to be an epiphenomenon of the complex interactions of the hypothalamus, the pituitary, the adrenal cortex and strongly mylenated neural fields, hard-wired to the reptilian brain for survival and reproductive purposes. Furthermore, the survival instinct in the patient is so strong that he has overridden the executive function of the neo-cortex with a deluge of delusional detritus and futile wish fulfillment. Aided by the latest medical breakthroughs in treatment of glioblastoma multiforme there is only a twenty percent likelihood that Mr. Ward may continue to survive the effects of his treatment for a statistical maximum of 1.3 years before recurrence of the cancer followed by an onslaught of drugs and the inevitable downward spiral to the **grave** — the point of no return, flat line, brain death, the worm farm. So long erstwhile "Osiris," hello extinction of consciousness. The prosecution rests.

Now, I rise to the defense with all the courage and conviction I can muster. I admit I was affected by the Decadron. But the effects rapidly diminished over a mere two and a half weeks, declining from the equivalent of five double espressos before bed to none. But I am certain of my experience of the Children of the Future. The feeling of the miraculous in everyday life and the sense of being blessed by this illness have steadily unfolded with enduring gratitude and conviction. Just to wake in the morning, and see the light on the trees and the sun in the blue sky has given me a most glorious feeling—I'm alive! I love my life. I do not fear death, having "died" already. Everything is so very new. My love for my family knows no bounds. The blessing of growing affection for friends and neighbors, far and near, has opened my heart. This inestimable gift I would not trade for anything.

Sane means both clean and sane. I had been washed clean, baptized.

Like those immersed by John in the Jordan, I, too, had a threshold experience; a "drowning" that loosened my etheric body from the physical. In that threshold state, what I saw changed me. My eyes opened.

As I returned to "normal," the muddy waters of first learning about my cancer had settled out. My priorities had clarified into just Being. The life-threatening nature of the illness receded for me into the background. For Andy, who was stoically carrying the emotional weight of the implications of my illness, such detachment was out of the question. But for me, immaculate Life remained. Restlessness became stillness. Uncertainty and fear turned to deep peace. Dark clouds and dust devils whirled away, leaving the clear blue sky.

FROM FUNK SHUI TO FENG SHUI

MY STUDY WAS A disaster area. Unanswered letters, heaps of unfiled documents, stacks of books, overcrowded shelves, useless mementos, articles to read, forms to fill, clutter, accumulated detritus of years, and things I might need someday. I was looking at illness. My formless, disorderly, proliferating tumor was reflected in the physical environment of my unpruned, chaotic, study. No wonder, I was glutted with the emanations of undealt-with stuff!

I told Margaret, my bath mistress, that I couldn't wait "to do battle" with the negative *elemental beings* lurking in my study and drive them from the field. She set me straight. "Nothing needs to be driven away. They just want to be recognized."

No matter what you may think about elemental beings—the wee folk, the elves that restore the poor cobbler and his wife to prosperity, or the Tomten who looks after the farm while the people sleep—a little appreciation of the unseen hands is called for if your study, attic, or basement look like mine.

Every horizontal surface had useless piles. The diagnosis was plain. The study was constipated, compacted. The free flow of energy was thwarted at every turn. I focused my newly liberated will for change on the study couch. What once had been a foldout bed for guests or slumber parties had become a self-storage container for stacks of useless information. We were being choked with catalogues, appeals, articles we were too busy to read, paperwork tasks undone, worthy causes junked, solicitations pending. The information glut was clogging the arteries. We were being mass marketed to death with consumer enticements we could not haul to the dump fast enough. We were on lists beyond our power to turn off, though we barely bought anything. How to turn off the porridge machine of useless drivel?

I focused my wrath on the threadbare couch and its "piles" (in the funkiest sense of the word). If the couch could be evicted from the study, the great constipation would be over and an excretion of years of buildup would ensue. Shortly after Thanksgiving the great catharsis would occur. The Doyles, Billy and his brothers, came with a pick-up truck. As Heracles diverted a river to muck out the Augean stables, here were the heroic Doyles to liberate this moribund couch from the study. With mover's finesse and brute force they maneuvered (or should I say manured) the couch out of the study, down the hall, and into the truck. The event was so important to me that I digitally recorded it for posterity, having been forbidden to lift anything greater than five pounds myself. This couch, "coincidentally" the size and weight of an Egyptian sarcophagus, I had invested with great symbolic meaning. This act would liberate creative energy, bring order out of chaos, free from prison the entombed Osiris, and set the *chi* flowing. Is that too much to expect? As I changed old habits in the study, my nascent tumor was put on notice that if it dared rear its Hydra head, I would chop it off with the sword of Feng Shui and burn the stump.

Soon after, Captain Buzz Buzz vacuumed the accumulated dust from all the books and shelves. I understand that a high percentage of household dust is sloughed-off skin. What the dust mites (with faces only a mother could love) don't consume floats in eternal descent in shafts of light and settles on every surface. Dust is us. It is a much-underrated natural resource, one hundred percent recyclable. In the body's economy, a tipping point is eventually reached where our power to regenerate new cells to replace the continuously dying epithelial cells is a losing battle that oceans of lotion cannot counteract. Whatever the proximate cause of one's demise, when the *life forces* leave the body, it quickly dissolves to the minerals that constituted it. "Ashes to ashes and dust to dust." This is not the case with the soul and spirit, which are dust-free. They are, however, encrusted with karma. Such reflections back my Feng Shui resolve with muscle. Cheerfully, I repainted the study at 8:00 p.m., an inconceivable hurdle before my illness.

Counter to this freeing of energy, as I've mentioned, I was being overwhelmed with an outpouring of good will and prayers flowing toward me. So much love. I could not just throw away these cards, children's pictures, poems, wise words, and heartfelt encouragement. Responding to more than a few was out of the question. I read them and put them in boxes, sorting out the most meaningful for future reference. It, too, was a Feng Shui problem: sorting essential from non-essential. How does one clear one's desk? The Napoleonic method is to let the correspondence pile up for weeks then, when much, if not all of it, has become obsolete, sweep it away in a single commanding gesture and start anew. Another alternative is to install a dumpster-compacter underneath the desk with a mechanical lever indicating "delete all." In my attempt to keep my mind clear, I still had a nagging doubt. Should I be cataloguing these names and addresses in some organized fashion for future acknowledgment? I came to answer, "No."

"No" has always been the hardest word for me to say. Advised by a friend, I have archived these cards in a special box, labeled "THE GIFT." Ultimately, no matter how we sort, all is destined for the compost heap. The relics of the past will molder away becoming the new soil. The new earth will put forth leaves of living green.

As I remained sequestered in the sanctuary of my house, I felt the numinosity of familiar objects illumined by my new lease on life. For example, for years a Saint Francis figure from New Mexico had been a familiar presence on the mantle. The simply carved *Santo* was missing a hand. I felt with a pang the missing hand as a symptom of my illness, the weakening of my will, that I had allowed years to go by without repairing it. Saint Francis was a gift from New Mexico I had given to my mother decades ago. It had returned to us at her death. It was saturated with meaning for me, since I once thought I would become a simple woodcarver myself. (I may yet.) Within the hour, I carved the hand and glued it on before going for our first interview with Dr. German to learn the results of the surgery. The maimed saint had his right hand restored. And I began to rediscover my own will.

MESSAGES

As I VACUUMED DUST from my books and library shelves, several powerful instances of synchronicity occurred. There was a beat-up old book of *The Adventures of Odysseus and the Tale of Troy* by Padraic Colum. As much as I appreciated this great storyteller's beautiful use of language, I already had a sufficient collection of the Greek epics and myths, and it was doubtful that I would teach again. Why should I keep this old thing? I had seen better copies for a buck in secondhand stores. Besides, I was intent on paring down my accumulated library and opening shelves for the new. Despite its wear and tear, instead of putting it into the recycling stack with my newly established executive authority, I took a peek inside. Hmmm...an inscription. "This is

Christy's book and I hope she will like it" (signed) Padraic Colum, January 14, 1919. It was a first edition given to the daughter of the poet Percy MacAye by his friend Padraic Colum. A thrill shot through me. Christy was perhaps ten years old at that time. She would go on to become a wonderful poet, speech artist, pioneer of the Rudolf Steiner School in New York City, inspiring teacher of literature, and wise woman. She had died a few years before this treasure resurfaced in my study.

Andy and I were proud to be friends of Henry and Christy Barnes. Christy had guided the festival life in Hawthorne Valley for years, and we were always a part of her speech choruses. She inspired us to love poetry and the spoken word. She taught Andy how to be the angel for the Middle English Coventry Christmas play, which we performed for years. A flood of memories of Christy's youthful wonder and enthusiasm rushed over me as I held her precious book in my hands, a birthday present given eighty-six years before from one lover of the Word to another. This moment of communion with someone who had died came as I faced the possibility of my own death. One of the speech choruses we would recite in honor of the departed for our All Soul's festival came back to me along with Christy's gestures, cadences, and *Schwung*:

> Spirits of your souls,
> Great active guardians,
> May your swinging wing strokes bring
> Our souls' entreating love
> To the human beings of the spheres
> Entrusted to your care.
>
> That united with your power
> Our entreaty stream with help
> To the souls whom lovingly we seek.
>
> *(Rudolf Steiner)*

I seek you, Christy. I feel you here, now.

The next numinous object to appear a few minutes later was a laminated card in my desk drawer, announcing the funeral of Zachary Culley. He had been my student for five years in my second class. He was a wonderful, Tom Sawyer kind of fellow, sunny and cheerful, strong and athletic. He had died tragically at age sixteen, missing his footing on the ledge rock above Strawberry Falls, the family swimming hole. He had taken to writing poetry and had given me a couple of his poems. One was clearly prophetic of his accidental death. His early death inspired me to compose a story weaving together threads of the Crusades, the search for the healing forces of the Holy Grail, a pilgrimage of redemption, and an urban garden in a down-and-out section of London. I would often think of Zachary and a young girl, Geneve, who was struck by a car at age seven, as this story unfolded within me over a period of months. Their deaths unleashed creative forces in me toward exploring the relationship of the living and the dead and spiritual guidance in time of need.

Cleaning out my desk brought the rush of strong remembrance of Zachary as I held his death announcement. Soon after, as I continued my Feng Shui sorting operation, determining which books to give to the school and which to keep, I opened a folk tale from Ethiopia, *The Miracle Child*. It was a story of deliverance and reunion. It was inscribed to Zachary, St. Nicholas Day, 1986! Zachary wanted to share the story with his classmates and had brought the book to school. I was flooded with memories of Zachary. I dug out a poem I had written for Zachary years ago, looking for clues of our deep connection. Now I hear it in his voice.

PILGRIMAGE

I have made a pilgrimage
beckoned by ringing bells,
reckoning the hours,
tolling all time tells.

I wound round the mystic maze
inlaid in sacred stones,
stood on the mute foundation
beneath the starry dome.

God grant me the grace,
I pray,
to ascend the tower stair,
guided by the still, small voice
breathed upon the air.

I see how lovingly the rose
with living light suffused,
reveals the sun in her embrace
with ever-shifting hues.

I stand before the altar
And kneel before the flame.
"Break bread with me, my brother."
He speaks who knows my name.

I am offered the holy cup,
my courage will not fail
to drink the water turned to wine
flowing from the Grail.

(For Zachary Culley, August 20, 1995)

Then came a message from Arvia. Arvia Ege had died in 1980. In the simple act of cleaning, she "appeared" to me inwardly. Arvia, along with her husband Karl Ege, Henry and Christy Barnes, Rudolf Copple, Fentress Gardner, and others were founders of Hawthorne Valley—the farm, the Visiting Students Program, and Hawthorne Valley School. Arvia, with Christy and Henry, had been founding teachers of the Rudolf Steiner School in New York City, the oldest Waldorf school in North America (1929), before dedicating their "retirement" to starting Hawthorne Valley in 1972. She had been a poet, sculptress, painter, and handwork teacher. She had also been present as a twenty-three-year-old at the Christmas conference of 1923, when Rudolf Steiner refounded the Anthroposophical Society out of the ashes of the first Goetheanum, destroyed by fire, New Year's Eve 1922–23.

My friend, Cecelia, brought soup as part of the Food Chain. She said, "Arvia wanted you to have this." Waves of electricity went through me. She handed over to me a six-inch plaster relief of an angel with the dove, the Holy Spirit, descending above her head. The plaque, shaped like a footprint, had traces of gold paint and was inscribed "PAX" — "peace." The angel gestured with her hand to her lips to be *silent*. I was dumbstruck. This message was so timely in stopping me from dissipating the power of the vision of the Children of the Future before it had time to ripen.

I had been inspired by Arvia's poetry, her vision of the possibilities for Hawthorne Valley, and her insight into the importance of Waldorf education for the future. The last few words of my last conversation with her were emblazoned on me, "…a servant of the Living Word." Now I held the work of her hands in mine, given through Cecelia, who had been very close to Arvia through the difficulties of the last two years of her life. "I've had this angel long enough," Cecelia said. "Now it's your turn." Again I felt the beneficent presence of the dead communicating with me that all will be well. That is not the same as a guarantee that I would live, but the whisper of hope that I am accompanied by a power of love and compassion that extend beyond my time on earth. PEACE and SILENCE — these would be my watchwords.

In the final push to clean out my desk, I came at last to a drawer that hadn't been opened for years. It was blocked by a clamped-on swing lamp and never used. Way at the back I was stunned to find a picture from fourth grade of my first class from 1980. I had a boy in my class named Eric Weitzman, whose father, a doctor, was dying of cancer at the time. He had a brain tumor. His wife and son and parents shared in the suffering, seeing the father's sharp decline. How could I help? We were studying Norse mythology as the language arts theme for the year, so I wrote a play called *The Death of Baldur,* intuiting that the wisdom and tragic beauty of the story would work therapeutically in this most difficult life situation. I cast Eric as the All-Wise Father, Odin, who would lose his son, the Sun god Baldur. As he was in fact losing his father in real life, I now looked at the photograph of Eric as Odin, a picture found by "chance," one that I had not seen in twenty-four years. I saw again with shocking vividness that Dr. Weitzman, deathly pale, had come to the play to see his son perform. A month later he had crossed the threshold. Now I also had a brain tumor, and later in the year would again see the fourth grade perform the same play I had written, beautifully led by their new teacher. But now the title to me would be *The Death and Resurrection of Baldur.* Eric-Odin whispered in his son Baldur's ear the "word of hope" that no one else one could hear.

As I regarded the picture of Eric, who experienced the loss of his father twenty-five years ago, I understood that my family and class and their parents were worried sick about my being taken by cancer. After we all realized I was in no position to continue teaching, my friend and fellow teacher Theo Lundin took on the class, though he was on sabbatical, trying to earn some money as a carpenter.

The wisdom of the Waldorf curriculum places the Norse myths on the cusp between early, "golden" childhood and the dramatic change of consciousness from wholeness and wonder toward greater separation and intellectuality. We were all going through a death experience, relinquishing the old consciousness with all its tragic beauty. Simultaneously, my guidance of and relationship to the class was being severed by iron circumstance. Even if it turned out that I should survive for now, everyone was in anxious suspense, forced to consider the prospect of my death. During my first meeting with Theo I urged him to do this play of death and resurrection. I knew *The Death of Baldur* was actually a healing balm for children of this age facing the reality of death. These lines from the play capture the gravity of this mood:

> **Goddesses:** Away sails our joy, away sails our light,
> Drifting to darkness, lost in the night.
> Away sails our hope, away sails our love,
> So sinks the sun from heaven above.

Odin: Yet in the darkness your light will shine,
Bringing joy, love, and hope to the land of the blind.

Aesir: Though you are distant, though you have died,
Shine in our hearts, our faithful guide,
Your truth and goodness drive away fear,
Though Day of Doom draws steadily near.
When we have crossed that fateful day,
We will see your face again we pray.

(song)

Bright Baldur sails the starlit sea
Bound for eternity,
His ship of light
Shines in the night,
Bearing Baldur's spirit bright.

Would Baldur's immolation be the fire of his resurrection?
Only Odin, the All-Wise, knew the secret word of hope.

Saint Nicholas

EVER SINCE THE EQUINOX, the light had been waning and the dark rising. Andy is a kindergarten teacher and the whole curriculum for a Waldorf kindergarten attunes itself to the cycle of the seasons in song, stories, pageants, and wonders. The school is also on a farm where the age-old reverence for the earth, the land, the life-giving power of the seeds, and the generous gifts of the cows and fellow creatures are a living reality, a daily practice. Starting with the date of surgery, Thursday, November 17, my illness unfolded into the increasing darkening of the year. An axial shift had occurred in my sense of time. I no longer had a daily teaching schedule where every minute was assigned. Except for doctors' appointments there was nowhere I had to be on time. I was living in wide-open, timeless space.

Still, time was marked by the seasonal festivals celebrated at Hawthorne Valley, tracking the passage of what was quite possibly my last year of life as the sun rose further and further south of east over the hills of the ridge line a few miles away. The harvest festival of Sukka passed me by. Halloween found the Riddle Master up a tree. A poignant melancholy rustled in the dead leaves. Ten days later I was diagnosed with cancer. For the first time I missed the Saint Martin's pageant and lantern walk on November 11. Brain surgery, November 17. Then came the Jewish New Year, Rosh Hashanah; followed by Yom Kippur, the solemn Day of Atonement, more meaningful than ever before. Judgment day was here. Then THANKSGIVING! Life! Harvest home. Advent—Light in the darkness. Saint Nicholas Day. Hanukkah—Festival of Light. Winter Solstice. Christmas—birth of the Holy Child. All these celebrations were lovingly, reverently reviewed, with the lighting of a candle of hope.

Saint Nicholas and Ruprecht came unexpectedly on the sixth of December to our house. In our seclusion, we had not expected any visitors, least of all a holy man. The white-bearded, blue-cloaked symbol of benevolence and generosity had made a special trip. Equally important, his silent companion, his servant and shadow, with his belt of chains, bag of apples, and lumps of coal accompanied him. Andy and I were dumbstruck with surprise and delight to be included on his rounds.

Historically, Nicholas, the Archbishop of Cusa, was known for his great generosity and compassion, especially toward children. He tirelessly helped the poor and the sick. He was also patron saint of sailors, guiding them safely to port from stormy seas. Stormy seas—that must be why he came to us, and also to remind me of the urgency of the Spirit of Generosity toward the Children of the Future. He had with him the Book of Life in which was inscribed the record of our deeds on pages light and dark. Our deeds, aspirations, resolves, and shortcomings witness the choices we make in life. "He knows when you are sleeping, he knows when you're awake, he knows if you've been bad or good, so be good for goodness sake."

We waited with utmost attention to hear his guiding wisdom in our exceptional circumstances. St. Nicholas spoke these words from the dark and light pages of the Book of Life:

ANDY

The only thing on your dark page
Is the darkness itself.
It will tell you only lies:
"NO WAY OUT,
GO BACK, GO BACK,
NO GOD, NO LIGHT,
ONLY BLACK."
DO NOT BELIEVE IT!
God sends his comforter...
A muse, a voice from deep within,
Dwell upon the truths,
Where the light begins!
The only thing on your light page
Is the light itself.
—HOLD THE LIGHT—
For you, for William, for us all.

WILLIAM

I see that you have not exactly been
Following doctor's orders:
—Are you resting enough?
—Are you letting visitors stay a little too long?
—Are you up all night doing God knows what?
I see also that you don't always listen
to your good wife. Do you?
She wants only the best for you.
Let her be your guardian and helpmate.
This will serve you well for today and
all your tomorrows.

If you can't sleep—get up—go out under the starry
    heavens.
At this blessed time, look up to find your home
in the unending stillness.
This you must do!!

And on the light-filled page.
Well what can I say?
So many entries...
Perhaps just this:
You have given all your love away,

And yet your heart is overflowing.
You have said all there is to say,
Without a thought of knowing.
You have done it all again today,
Loving, Knowing, Doing, Growing.

GOD BLESS YOU WILLIAM
SHINE ON....

Ruprecht gave us each a golden nut and an apple. For me the
nut was the golden gift of my life-changing illness. And the apple
was straight from the Tree of Life.

Ruprecht was serving the saint as penance for past misdeeds.
According to legend he was mute because his tongue had been cut
out by the authorities for telling lies, a bit draconian for modern
sensibilities. Nicholas had compassion for Ruprecht, our shadow
self, carrying the sooty encrustation of karma. This is like Marley's ghost from *A Christmas Carol* dragging the chains he forged
in life. Ruprecht and I are working our respective karmas off, serving one who stands for us as witness, guide, friend, and comforter.
In time the soot falls away, we are washed clean, and become our
true selves bearing gifts for the Children of the Future.

As Ruprecht left, he dropped a cabbage that thumped on the
floor and rolled to my feet. Magically-comically the implications
as I read them were, don't let yourself become a cabbage head,
overwhelmed by vegetative abundance. Make soup and slaw and
get on with life.

St. Nicholas delivered a message from me to my class, December 6, 2005. This was ghost written by me as I had always done before. Don't tell anyone. From the Book of Life:

GIFTS

On the day of your birth
You were given gifts,
The seeds of your own will,
To sow upon the earth,
That through your work
The seeds might grow
Into a fruitful garden,
Protected by the Tree of Life
Whose branches hold up heaven.

Now your roots grip solid ground,
Glad to be alive.
Your head bears a golden crown
Like the sun that lights the sky.
Your breath weaves in and out
Like the ocean tides,
As the fountain of your heart
Sings the song of life.
You crossed the rainbow bridge,
You left your heavenly home
To walk the green, fruitful earth
Beneath the starry dome.
You know this is the place
To give all your gifts away,
Scattering them like golden seeds
Unfolding every day.
Seed-deeds ripen beneath the sun
Rooted in fertile will
To become the Bread of Life
When the seeds are milled.

We will break bread together
At the Thanksgiving Feast
Where the bounty of all your gifts
Is gathered in at last.
Take hands, dear family,
All my sisters and my brothers,
Let's give thanks that we are here
To learn from one another.
We are all completely different
On our own and apart,
Yet one is our humanity,
In the Sunshine of the heart.
Few can say what gift one bears
While it is just a sprout,
It takes hard work, rain, and sunlight
To let the gift come out.
But then it shows for all to see
As radiant as a flower
That opens wide to the light,
Fulfilled through its power.

So ask yourself,
"What is my gift,
How can I help it grow?"
One day you'll reap the harvest
From the seeds today you sow.

It was surprising to me that, in the throes of illness, the well-springs of poetry were flowing again. It was imperative that I tap deeper sources if I were to survive my illness. But whether or not I would still be around, I could foresee the abundant harvest that would be gathered in by such children as these, so awake to their will to work in a new way for the future.

During the Advent season, the four weeks preceding Christmas, we had daily visits. The Food Chain, delivering us our evening meal, meant we would have an hour to sit by the fire together with a colleague or a family from my class. This contact was tremendously healing for us. The warmth of mutual affection had burst into flame because of my illness. In the ordinary course of life there had been little opportunity to socialize during this festive season, but now that I was seriously ill and feeling great at the same time, we found time to be with one another, laugh, have tea, tell stories. The hearth fire burned brightly with seasoned oak delivered by fellow teachers Martin Ping, Gary Ocean, Nick Francischelli, and the fifth graders. And the FOOD! We ate like royalty. Every evening there was a wonderful home-cooked meal with all the trimmings. We couldn't keep up with the delicious leftovers before there was another knock at the door. When the hour was up, the family or friend would leave. Hugs all around. And Andy and I would light the Advent candle, the light that shines in the darkness of winter. We would hold hands, give thanks to God, for family, friends, and food. We were partaking of the daily bread of life. So much to live for. Life!

In this mood of deep gratitude, I wrote my class and their parents an Advent poem:

ADVENT

Held
in the circle
of your love
a child is born
today!
He looks
on earth
from Heaven above
in the singing
Milky Way.

– – –

Time rolls round
to come back down
and place his feet
on solid ground,

So he descends
the rainbow bridge
into his Mother's arms
who wraps him
with the sunlight
and protects him
from all harm.
How good to be
on earth again
beneath the Sacred Tree
where you and I
learn and grow
into God's mystery.

UNIVERSAL HEALTH CARE

Uncertainty about the future created bedrock certainty of the value of the present. All that had been ordinary and timeworn was now precious and new. Simple things: the red winter sunset over the blue ridge of the Catskills, the toasty fire, the silence, the peace, afternoon tea, chicken soup on the stove, a letter from a friend, a Food Chain visit, blessing the meal while holding hands with Andy, star gazing at the winter sky, inspirational reading before bed, coziness, dreamland.

I had been given the gift of *time*. In the twinkling of an eye my life took a turn from every moment spoken for with an ever-increasing backlog of tasks…to simple Being. I was not in denial about my future. The fact of death sooner or later was not a question. How one related to death was a huge question. Let walls of DENIAL erected to defend oneself from fears of abandonment, annihilation, extinction, and the cold void dissolve like ice in spring. Cancer speeds the process of discerning what is important from what is not. There are two interwoven paths to traverse: "I am in a fight for my life against cancer," or "Cancer, teach me what I need to learn to change my life, I resolve to work with you." As necessary as it was to combat cancer by every means, I sensed that it was equally true that wise guidance lay hidden among the thorns.

I believed I had had an experience of coming attractions. My strong conviction was that my moment of crossing had been put on hold. I felt a strong but undefined sense of purpose in my new life. Cancer would collaborate with me in the inner and outer tasks still needed to fulfill my life's work.

I had been blessed in my choice of vocation as a class teacher, equal parts challenging and rewarding. Though I missed the children, there was no way I could ever take up teaching children again. That requires more time than I had, great stamina, ego strength, and resolve. What teaching children required had once sustained me; now the demands would have been life-threatening for me. No, my new job was first to transform all old habits. This would effect changes right through the cells of my body. This decisive reversal, from out-flowing expenditure of energy for others to receiving help for myself, could not have been more dramatic. From here on my priority must be my own healing.

Mobilization. The post-surgery team:

Dr. Susan Weaver, my neuro-oncologist at Albany Medical Center, would be the cancer specialist consulting with us, advising and prescribing treatment; Dr. Kim, radiologist, Cavel Cancer Treatment Center, would supervise the radiation treatments; Dr. Margaretha Hertle, general practitioner, Ita Wegman Clinic, would oversee the Iscador therapy and prescribe, in consultation with Dr. Thomas von Rottenburg, oil essences for oil dispersion bath therapy; nurse Margaret Rosenthaler would administer oil dispersion bath treatment; nurse Phyllis Talbott would administer Iscador infusions; Jane Wright, physical therapist and intuitive healer, would provide ongoing rebalancing; Sidney Fulop, Jungian analyst, would provide weekly counseling; Lee Cheek, Rosen Body Work massage therapist, would provide periodic massage support; Zeev Kolman, bioenergetic healer; Nicole Furnee, rhythmic massage; Gili Lev, music therapy. Enough already! Wait, there's more...Dan and Jack (love your phlebotomists) for blood tests every other week. Three cheerful radiation technicians; Nurse Betty; Lindsay and Jorita, prescriptions and appointments; my drivers to the Cavel Center or Albany Med: Andy, Leif, Pancho, Larry, Christiana and Frank Wall, Sidney, Pamela, Dan. That's twenty-eight people so far looking after little Bill. Throw in three more receptionists, four anonymous lab technicians, five insurance representatives (Unum, CDPHP, TIAA-CREF, HVA, GENEX), two financial consultants, and a partridge in a pear tree. Let's not forget the twelve people involved with my surgery and hospital stay. The count so far is fifty-four people who were part of this shepherding process through an incredibly complex labyrinth. Later on, in Switzerland, I attended two clinics and came into contact with another twelve doctors and therapists who were on my case. Some people monitor their health with blood cell counts. I track the therapist to biomass ratio (T/BM).

Except for my friends who drove me to these places, giving me profound advice and support every mile of the way, all these people were health care professionals—courteous, cheerful, funny, attentive, dedicated, punctual, efficient, and kind. I am awed by this network of humanity devoted to caring for others. Whatever criticism I may have of the one-sidedness of our health care-insurance-pharmaceutical systems, I was privileged to be the recipient of incredibly humane treatment on every hand. May the gaping holes in our health care systems be repaired. I cannot account for the fact that I was lifted up to receive all this care. I am deeply grateful for the grace I have received. Thankfulness shall be my path. I can only pray that everyone—the poor, the cold, the hungry, the destitute, the aged, the demented, the chronically ill may also receive the warmth of human compassion that I experienced. Let the warmth of gratitude and mercy, the circle of giving and receiving, unceasingly, compassionately flow through us as the life stream of humanity.

I'm terminally ill (not departing yet, of course, but ultimately) and want to contribute my two cents toward a healthier tomorrow. My appreciation for the help I have been receiving takes me quite beyond myself to think BIG.

Zoom out from one isolated individual, self-important me, to envision the Archetype of all humanity in holy wholeness. Each of us is one unique cell in that vast embracing body of humanity. Picture that mighty being completely healthy and balanced. Now picture the pain and suffering we see everyday rising all over the globe. This is a wound borne by humanity within the Universal Human Being. We ask this cosmic being, "What ails thee, brother?" Now, in asking, the same light, life, and love that are the separate droplets of our compassion for one another begins to flow wherever there is need. Healing waters lave every limb and permeate every cell. The Spirit of the World offers the cup of healing to all who thirst. The three billion living soul-cells join the choirs of angels and the revered ancestors in a cosmic Medicine Wheel encompassing with love and gratitude this ailing macrocosmic Human Being.

This is already a galactic-scale operation, but, fortunately, we have more disk space in our Imagination hard drive. Our project is big, but doable. Every human being (no child left behind) harnesses her or his guiding star (guardian angel) for the healing cause. Our united will for healing, our focused love, will restore and rejuvenate each wounded soul, each part of the whole. Many members, one body. Only when you are healed may I too become whole. Only when your sorrow becomes my sorrow, your joy becomes my joy, does the body of the world find balance, harmony, and healing.

Each of the cells/selves of the circling Medicine Wheel in the wisdom of this mighty body knows what to do to bring about a great miracle. Imagine rank upon rank of the army of healers—Dr. Schweitzer is there, and so is Mother Teresa, as heavenly inspirers, all the more effective for having crossed the threshold; all the sisters of mercy swell the throng; the Red Cross, the Red Crescent, Doctors Without Borders, the Salvation Army fan out in support; UNICEF, UNESCO, UNAMEIT are on board; Sloan-Kettering, Mt. Sinai, Dana-Farber, Cedar-Sinai, Saint Peter's, Saint Luke's, and all hospitals and clinics join the chorus; shamans of the world unite hand in hand with the World Wide Wiccan Web; the Healing Harmonies marching band of music therapists contribute "Ode to Joy" with a 50,000-voice choir accompanied by gamelan and steel drum bands; African drumming of all tribes sets people dancing in the street until the rhythms reach down to the core of the Great Mother's singing, swaying benevolent body.... Humanity's Immune System is on the march, circulating with healing will to the cold, hungry, imprisoned (that's everyone), naked, and ill in every country, serving life and honoring death. The Holy Comforter and the Mother of Mercy, by whatever name you know them, come to your bedside, come to my bedside, offering the cup of healing to every child, woman, and man. Now the Universal Human Being, the one in the center of the Medicine Wheel, radiant with the love coursing through every cell of the great body, is made whole and the mission of Love, the mission of the Earth, is fulfilled!

I know what you are thinking. Is this practical? Or...Utopian, demented, off the wall, no way, poppycock, consult your pharmacologist, bipolar, ludicrous, pie-in-sky, la-la land, unrealistic, quixotic, dream on, etcetera. I never said this would be easy. Just bear with me while I address the major issues that oppose such a historic shift. The immediate task is to envision a human-to-human compassion jihad-crusade-mission dedicated to overcoming thirst, hunger, poverty, illness, homelessness. How can I help you, Everyman? Bless those legions already living their lives in selfless service. From now on, your needs come before mine. You and I are one, I am you, you are me. "Where love is, God is also." Now, for this to work, a Concord of Altruism will be drawn up by unanimous consent for our collective signature. Mission: healing a wounded world and healing ourselves in the process. There are three boxes to check on your ballot: giver, receiver, or giver/receiver. Check all three. You are free to sign. From this moment forward there will be an axial shift of priorities. The tide is turning. The annual resources of the collective military-industrial-complex will be reallocated to the aforementioned mission. Nations will cooperate to become economic engines of humanitarian aid and global *philanthropy*. The *spirit of generosity*, wanting only the best for humankind, has agreed to simultaneously inspire governments, billionaires, captains of industry, peace activists, religious leaders, the custodians of the natural resources of the world, and everyone who subscribes to the Golden Rule of all religions to study war no more, cap corporate and shareholder profits at a level that allows for the creation of a superfund of generosity, eliminate usury, forgive debt, redistribute the wealth, tithe, equitably apportion resources according to need, and change ourselves from the perpetuation of "enlightened self-interest" to "enlightened selflessness." We can do this. We just have to change all our habits.

This is what I have to do also if I am to eliminate terrorist cancer cells, fear, and imbalances of all kinds from my own body.

OK. We're agreed then. Altruism, it's not just a good idea, it's a cosmic law. The debate is over and the fine points took much less time than I thought. We are of one mind. In the spirit of potlatch s/he who gives the most away gets no cash prize. The joy of giving is its own reward. But you will receive the undying gratitude of all those you have helped and their aid when it's your turn to receive. Our "Treasures in Heaven" reward program will offer advance credit for your next incarnation (if you earned it). Everyone you helped will help you in your next life. The law of karma will ensure complete compliance. You thought if you got to "heaven" you just stayed there for eternity? Sorry, that is a fundamental misunderstanding of the mission of Love on earth. That would be an egoistic "pursuit of happiness," a "health and wealth" illusion. No, my brothers and sisters, we have a larger task before us. UNIVERSAL HEALTH CARE. We can reach the goal when we see God in Everyman.

❧

Where was I? Yes, the human face of health care. What I was privileged to receive required the cooperation of sixty-six highly educated and trained people. They in turn are supported by a less visible but equally necessary network of members, including custodians, cooks, parking lot attendants, administration, reception, you name it, they have it. Now most of these people have no health benefits. Of the five thousand employees at Albany

Medical Center many have no health insurance. We know that about forty-eight million people in this great land of ours have no health care insurance. We are aware that family and business budgets are breaking over rising insurance and medical costs. We also know that doctors are abandoning the profession because of paperwork, malpractice insurance, and pressure to see more patients on a rigid schedule determined by the bottom line. The complexities of fixing the system and ushering in UNIVERSAL HEALTH CARE boggle the mind of all but the most determined wonks. People become comatose or switch the channel if anyone wades into this thicket to "clarify" the intractable issues. There is leaden inertia, stupefaction, and gridlock with such massive hurdles to be surmounted. And the bugaboo fear of socialized medicine. Ohhhh, save me! Let "free market" forces handle health care? Ha!

Meanwhile, I'm getting medical insurance and eight MRIs per year to keep me alive for another few months. OK, maybe I'll get off for good behavior and live a while longer just to demonstrate how it's done. But really, we don't need so many gadgets when people are hungry and thirsty.

I'm a simpleton, but it seemed transparently criminal to me when big pharma and Brown and Root, Halliburton, et al get *carte blanche* construction contracts during the Iraq war with negligible fiscal accountability. That inspires *impotent outrage*. The energy lobby and oil company CEOs collude with Dick Cheney to write energy policy that becomes law. I smell a rat. *Impotent outrage*. Oil companies reap record-breaking profits from the high costs of energy and get to keep the money to help us become less dependent on foreign oil. Give me a break. *Impotent outrage*. Hundreds of millions thrown at Katrina are unaccounted for and the poor become homeless refugees. *Impotent outrage*. Fannie May restates its earnings (read losses) by ten billion dollars, admitting no culpability. *Impotent outrage*. CEO salaries rise through the stratosphere to a 451 to 1 ratio compared with an average worker's share. Excessive wealth becomes concentrated in the hands of the top one percent of the population. The promiscuous growth of the national debt falls into the same maelstrom of untamable beasts. *Impotent outrage.* I better go shopping to help the economy?

The gesture of the "unseen hand" is always the same. It is an obscene gesture. The beast grins over its brood of voracious, like-minded predators and special interests who exploit complex systems with labyrinthine schemes, arcane language, and lies for power and personal gain. The hydra-headed "greed is good" dragon stalks the land. Unbridled competition, survival of the fittest, me-first are crocodile values. Cold-blooded, heartless, reptilian consciousness is colonizing brains with selfish Machiavellian schemes. Will human ideals, not animal instincts, subdue the dragon? Will brotherhood-sisterhood, service, cooperation, and compassion re-inspire our economic life? Stay tuned.

Meanwhile, no wonder I feel ill. Do I allow myself to choke on impotent rage? Or do I just shrug it off, shake my head, and say, "There's nothing I can do. That's just how it is"? Maybe I'll buy more body armor. But I can't turn off the drumbeat of Improvised Exploding Devices detonating in my inner ear. Insurgency cells are competing for territory in the back alleys and contorted convolutions of the Baghdad of my mind. My cellular receptors are on red alert. *I have cancer!* Meanwhile, an acid rain of bad news and noise pollution is corroding my homeland security defense system. Pieces of men, women, and children of all faiths and colors are flying through the fiery virtual air. My negative thoughts and fears are feeding the beast. The slaughter of the innocents. *Impotent outrage.*

I must enter the quiet zone. Peace. Solitude. Let me drink from the Sacred Fountain.

OPEN DOOR

MY CANCER WAS SYMPTOMATIC of being out of harmony. Way out. I needed a tuneup. All systems had taken a prescribed beating from radiation and chemotherapy. With my full consent, the death forces had fulfilled their mission and stopped the regeneration of cancer cells at least for the moment. That's just the way it is. Once cancer has been detected and dealt with to the best of modern medicine's ability, the patient has become a "survivor!" Images of the Holocaust arise. The emaciated survivors with their shaved heads and hollow-eyed stare. Are we in a long, slow Death Camp of some kind? Are we an inferior race with a genetic flaw, unacceptable customs and beliefs, bearing the burden of some secret stigma, branded by a malevolent Führer? Or is it precisely in the Shadow of Death that the spirit self flames up and illumines the darkness for oneself and others?

Notable among the cancer patients I have met, some in grievous pain, there are several who have said, "This illness has been a blessing to me." Of those who have remained quiet about their illness, at least to me, one nonetheless feels in their silent struggle a radiant courage to go through the cleansing fire. Depth psychologists Robert Sardello and Cheryl Sanders describe spiritual courage in facing cancer in their introduction to *Iscador:*

> Through the practical spirituality of courage we develop a kind of double vision. The ordinary realm of perception, feeling, thinking, and action goes on, but everything in these modes of experience is also seen as corresponding to something of a spiritual nature. This spiritual intensification can see us through the most difficult trials imaginable.

Cancer engages body, soul, and spirit—in the Holy of Holies of the "I am." Outside intervention goes only as far as the courtyard of the Temple. Transformation is needed at the cellular level; the level of one's thoughts, feeling, and will; and

at the level of one's deepest, as yet unknown spiritual intentions
for this life.

Engaging one's illness is a labyrinth. The man-eating Mino-
taur awaits its human prey in the core of the maze. Theseus, the
hero, courageously enters the labyrinth to prevent the continuing sacrifice of the flower of youth to the beast within. This we
must do individually if the monster is ever to be overcome. Theseus receives magical help. The King's daughter has provided
a slender golden thread that can lead him out again from that
dark descent and confrontation with annihilation back into the
light of day. Emerging from this conflict, the hero has achieved
the power to free all those who had lived in fear of the beast.
What is this golden thread? It is the light that shines in the
darkness.

We all harbor cancer cells. The integrated unity of the "I"
with the immune system harmonizes cellular growth in service
to the whole body. Dr. Friedrich Lorenz eloquently underscores
this polarity between cell and organism in *Cancer: A Mandate to
Humanity:*

> Cellular pathology and cellular physiology are under a mis-
> conception when they designate the cell as the basis of all
> life and regard the human organism merely as a conglom-
> eration of cells. The truth is that the human being is seen to
> be a totality, in relation to the cosmos, and constantly bat-
> tling with the separate existence of the cells. In reality, it is
> the cell which constantly disturbs our organism instead of
> building it up.
>
> It is in the nature of the cell to maintain a separate exis-
> tence. It must be constantly modified and differentiated
> to perform the organism's tasks and goals. By serving the
> organism, the cell must sacrifice its own separate existence.
> Only then will it become a true organ cell.
>
> It is not the cells in their growth which regulate the func-
> tions of the organism but rather the organism which takes
> hold of the cells and designates their functions.

Cellular growth is regulated by formative forces. The unity of the "I" and the immune system recognizes and eliminates what is alien and inimical to the human archetype, in this case the uninhibited growth of cancer. One cannot remain a passive recipient of treatments at the hands of dedicated doctors and technicians and hope to live. You have to take hold and engage the illness. Jacob wrestles with the angel all through the night. He will not let go until he receives the angel's blessing. Even when the angel dislocates Jacob's hip (essential to balance), he continues to grapple with the divine being. At dawn he wrests a blessing from his angelic adversary.

This courage to persevere against the odds may not seem possible to one living with pain and fear. But I know it is. I have seen this flame in others and received it myself. For love of a friend or for yourself, you can turn toward the light any moment you will yourself to do so: I am alive, I am attentive to this precious moment with you, I welcome the tender mercies and minor miracles of the day. My door is open to you my new friend, my brother, my sister, my unknown Self. Today, if I can find the words, I will tell you how much I love you. If words fail, my eyes still will tell you what you already know. If my eyes are closed, simply hold my hand, and I will feel your heart and you mine. I am with you.

In this moment of presence, just now, writing the word *door* opened the door of a memory of Annemarie, Dr. Philip Incao's* wife, who died of cancer fifteen years ago. I vividly recall the fall's blazing glory the October of her death. She loved color and permeated her home with beauty. In tribute to her approaching death, autumn had never been as clear, brilliant, and poignant as that year. The warm days and clear nights lingered and seemed a celebration of her life and imminent crossing. No one could blame her for not wanting to leave this glory, not knowing what awaited her on the other side. I still feel her hand in mine as we shared a silent farewell on my last visit. This poem came to me on the breath of her vivid presence two weeks before her passing. I see her now:

---

*   Dr. Philip Incao, a shining star of anthroposophic healing, now practicing anthroposophic medicine in Colorado, was the founding physician of the medical clinic that serves our school and valley.

OPEN DOOR

No need to knock,
The door is open wide.
You know you're always welcome,
Won't you come inside?
You will find me here to greet you
With the feast for all prepared.
To celebrate our friendship,
Fall's fire is everywhere...
Our table is the earth itself,
The cloth, the meadows green.
Star candles burn above,
Our wine the flowing stream.
Our hearth fire is the blessed sun,
Sunlight our daily bread,
Lifting dancing daisies white,
Raising roses red...
Feel free to come here anytime,
You need never feel alone.
If you seek a true friend,
I am always here at home.
You know, I will never love you less,
I can only love you more,
For nothing stands between us
When you walk through my door.

Three weeks later, she had crossed over. I took a long walk soon after and strongly felt Annemarie's guiding presence. The beauty of the fall was again the doorway to silent communion with my friend.

When I am still
I find you there,
Along the forest way.
Peaceful light,
Clear as air,
Fairer than the day.

"What do you see?"
Your eyes beseech.
"Only falling leaves."
"Come deeper then,"
You beckon,
"There's so much else to see."

I try to follow
Where you lead
With step so swift and light,
When I pause,
You are there
In the heart of quiet.

"What do you hear?"
You ask without a word.
"Only the passing of the wind,
The call of a frightened bird."

"Come further then, still further in,
The music is so near,
So deeply, joyfully it sounds
Even stones can hear."

She led me to the mountain stream,
She bathed my eyes
And quenched my thirst,
She woke me from my shadow dream
And led me to the rocky verge...
And freed me like a swallow
To fly as light as light,
Born aloft upon the breath
Of self-sustaining grace
From the rock-bound world below
To the boundless blue of space.

"Now may you see,"
She spoke to me,
"Whose rays embrace the earth

That the body's dying seed
May spring to spirit birth,
Uplifted by the sun's fire
Whose gold flame burns away
Shadow, sorrow, loss, desire
In the dawning day;
Until by light
I am made light,
And I through love arise
To find my Self among the stars
Whose radiance never dies."

She went on,
And I returned
Unto the holy ground
The rocks, the trees,
The fallen leaves,
The ever-living now.

Now, with cancer's clairvoyance, I see this poem was written for Annemarie for All Soul's Day, November 11, 1991, the same week as my diagnosis, surgery, and out-of-body experience fourteen years later. The veil between worlds again had parted.

My conviction was that an open door of spiritual help was there for me as it is for all who seek it. From my current vantage point, I don't rule out that I was already being prepared by wise guidance for my own meeting with cancer these many years later. With such a friend as Annemarie, why would I feel sad then or now? Her helping hand reaches toward me tenderly from the farther shore. I feel her hand in mine after these many years as we shared our last good-bye. In my life she was a forerunner in facing cancer with courage. Now it is my turn to face cancer and to reach my hand to others.

How can the suffering patient find the fountain of spiritual courage to meet cancer? "Ask and it shall be given. Knock and the door shall open." Immerse yourself in the waters of life. "What if I can't swim? I am afraid."

The river of grace will hold you up. Your body is light.

Call me and I will hear you, care for you, soothe you, commune with you, help you, lift you up, give you water, nourish you, stand vigil, pray for you, guard you, guide you, receive you, give you strength, give you joy, grant you peace, lead you. I come when you call.

❧

During my senior year in high school, 1964, my senior English teacher, the mysterious Mr. Fremd, kept a "Montividean jackass urger" in his desk. Very rarely but strategically, he would whack the bone-handled leather strap across his desk like a crack of thunder. He said many enigmatic things that year. A door slammed down the hall and he said, hand cupped to his ear, "That's the saddest sound in the world." He played Mendelssohn's first violin concerto for us and said, "If you listen closely to this you will understand the whole 'calculus of pleasure and pain.'" We discovered only later that it was the last year of his life. He was dying of cancer and none of us knew it. In my yearbook, he wrote, "*Ora pro nobis.*" Pray for us. I thought it was only a football cheer.

Three years later, the summer of 1967, summer of Peace and Love, I had a powerful experience of his presence one night. I had hitchhiked to Alaska and was returning when I saw against the starry sky, on a cosmic scale, the smiling, ethereal faces of Mr. Fremd and Fred Walker, a close high school friend who had died in a car accident two years before. The night stars shone right through their transparent countenances. It was as though they were singing: "We are fine, death is nothing to fear, all is well."

I believed them. Now more than ever.

SHOW-ME-THE-MONEY MEETS ANGELS OF GENEROSITY

RECENTLY A FRIEND GAVE me a small tin box of peppermints. A year had passed since my cancer outbreak. Meaning is in the air. I have inklings of signs, foreshadowings, premonitions, and Janus-headed enigmas that could illuminate my past and provide clues to the future in the twinkling of an eye. What had once been amusing whimsy could catapult me to thrilling revelation. The banal had been lifted into the imaginary. Taken-for-granted objects, forgotten books, old photographs, etcetera were appearing in my life as golden keys or riddles to be deciphered. Being broadcast to me was a language of inexplicable numinosity that defied logic and rational explanation, implying instead wise intention. I think many people have such experiences, but if one is staring at the statistical likelihood of death within a year, such clues are no longer curious and amusing but become powerfully significant. I casually looked at the picture on the cover of the peppermint tin — the Alps (before long I would be transported there). The mints were "St. Claire's." Hmmm... my daughter's name. "Deliciously potent." Then I opened the tin. This quotation appeared.

> Before you speak, listen.
> Before you write, think.
> Before you spend, earn.
> Before you invest, investigate.
> Before you criticize, wait.
> Before you quit, try.
> Before you retire, save.
> Before you die, give.
> *William A. Ward*

William A. Ward — hey, that's my name! I am receiving counsel directly pertinent to my situation through a tin of mints! How do they do that? Who are *they*? Meaningful coincidence, synchronicity, numinous objects; however you classify such communications, my gooseflesh indicator raised the hairs of my arm. The inscription on the tin is a distillation of life wisdom pithy enough to be an epitaph. Who is this William A. Ward guy? I bet he's a relative. I'm in the throes of financial decisions, maybe I should look up William, my alter ego, as a personal financial advisor. Key words speaking so specifically to my current status make me feel like I have been personally handed a map. "Listen," "think," "write," "earn," "investigate," "invest," "save," "retire," "give."

But how could I passively trust these potentially random signs in the stream of life? I needed to control what was hopelessly adrift. How to handle financially an illness this serious was a daily concern. It had to be managed. What shape would Andy be left in if I, God forbid, succumbed to the illness? Where was the money going to come from to pay for alternative medicines? What was the annual burn rate of our resources? What insurance coverage did we have? What was the limit on our home equity line of credit? How was our monthly budget affected by my "early retirement" from teaching? Funeral expenses? Insult to injury. Could I withdraw without penalty from my retirement savings for medical expenses? What was the magnitude of medical expenses we could claim as deductions from our taxes? What did our disability insurance cover? Was I eligible for Social Security Disability benefits? Welcome to the Fund Fun House.

My first investment toward answering these pressing questions was in a mechanical pencil. I had ledger forms. Rachel Schneider had already volunteered to help Andy deal with the intricate bureaucratic complexities of medical insurance, co-pays, time lags, form filing, the backing and forthing that dealing with hospitals, drug providers, and insurance companies requires in triplicate. Paper, legalese, miscommunication, red tape, and automated systems with categories that don't fit your questions formed a labyrinth from which there was no escape. "This call is being monitored for quality control...all our service representatives are currently occupied. Your call will be answered in the order it was received...press 1 for claims...2 for account status...3 for billing...4 for going postal...5 to repeat the options...6 for a pleasant robotic voice that says 'I didn't quite get that'...7 to be put on permanent hold...8 and you'll have ten seconds to punch in your claim number, your insurance provider code, your pin, Social Security, and claim numbers, followed by the # key...9 if you're unsure of any of these numbers and would like to be told to call back during business hours with the correct information.... If you would like to revert to the main directory to hear these options again, please scream at the top of your lungs.... If you would like to release your tenuous hold on life, you may do so by pressing the eject button at any time."

Andy had always been our family accountant and had once worked in the days of pencil and paper for a hospital in the insurance/bills/accounting area. What goes around, comes around. Rachel, the farmer's wife, was a key figure in the Hawthorne Valley Association with a great deal of experience in public relations, planning, and communications. As karma would have it, Rachel and Andy and I had been friends and students together at the Waldorf Institute of Adelphi University thirty years ago. Here she was now to help us out. Small world.

Memories of my father sitting at his desk with his mechanical pencil on his day off, getting his books up to date, came back to me. As a child, I was mystified by Dad's behavior. Now I was in his chair budgeting, projecting retirement income scenarios, plotting variable rates of growth, and reading the fine print of opaque insurance policies. The goal was to ensure that, in the event of my untimely demise, Andy would be, as my father and father-in-law would have said, "well situated," aside from the incalculable loss of her life's partner. My father had conveyed to me that one never talked openly about politics, religion, or money. That was "not done." I am making an exception here, Dad, now that I have some idea how the best-laid plans can turn on a dime.

I have always had a very unusual relationship to money. My father and mother grew up during the depression. That left an indelible scar. His father never regained his financial footing and the habit of thrift ran deep. Parting with money for a new car was postponed year after year. Taking on any debt was out of the question. Home mortgage payments always came first. Brother Dave and I had savings accounts from the earliest age, an allowance, piggy banks, and coin collections. One of Dad's great regrets was handing in silver and gold for paper money in the 1930s as required by law. He kept close watch on the stocks of local companies National Standard (his employer), Clark Equipment, and Kawneer Company.

When I was ten or twelve, Dad had set up each of us with a hundred shares of National Standard Company as a hedge against inflation, held for us by him in trust. He encouraged us to keep track of the stocks through our local paper. He himself kept track religiously with a ledger book of dividends for Dave and me. I admired his engineering draftsman's clarity as he wielded his mechanical pencil to keep the wolf from the door with spells of dates and numbers ritually recorded. But I wondered why he wasn't outside playing.

One of my earliest and most significant memories in relationship to money occurred on a Christmas visit to Chicago to see the astounding, mechanically animated store windows of the Marshall Fields department store, with gnomes and Santa's elves preparing for Christmas (the retailers' pot of gold). When it was time to go back home to Niles, Michigan, we were walking down the New York Central train platform to catch the Twentieth Century Limited. It was cold as only the Windy City can be. I reached up to hold my father's hand. I'd guess I was four or five years old. A soldier came walking straight toward me. There was no getting around him. He must have been on Christmas leave. He stopped in front of me, bent over with a father's kindness, and put a shiny quarter into my hand. I looked up at my Dad to see whether I could keep this treasure. Dad shook his head, "No." I sadly offered it back, remembering we don't accept gifts or candy from strangers. Why, I wasn't sure. The soldier knelt down to my level, looked me in the eye and benevolently smiled. "Keep it or I'll break your arm," he said gently. He closed my fingers around the shiny quarter. The coin was mine. "Merry Christmas."

That moment made the deepest impression on me. It was like the fairy tale of the star money, which falls from heaven for the poor orphan girl who is lost in the woods. This sense of being mysteriously and freely rewarded, not by dint of effort, but by grace, was sharply reinforced six years later. It was the fifth grade bake sale, Bill Ward solo cashier. After a few customers there was a lull. I counted the change to see how the bake sale was going. Oh, my God! There has been a terrible mistake. Someone has given me a rare old penny in change. I know my pennies. I habitually bought rolls of them from the bank searching for old ones to add to my collection. This coin was a very rare 1909 S. (San Francisco) penny, the first year Lincoln head pennies replaced the old Indian head pennies. Only a quarter million of these had been minted. My little boy's collector's heart (baseball cards, football cards, stamps, coins, chestnuts, fossils, minerals, insects, and butterflies) was pounding. "Mrs. Watson! Look what I found! A 1909 S. VDB in good condition. I'm sure it was given to the bake sale by mistake. We have to find out who gave it so we can give it back." This would not concern the investors of today. That's when I realized that I didn't know whether it had the maker's initials, VDB, on the obverse or not. My heart sank. It was worth either $10.00 or $250. I turned it over. In the tiniest letters the designer's initials were there. I blinked to make sure I wasn't seeing things. "I'm sorry Bill, but there isn't any way we can find who gave that to you among all those pennies. You'll just have to keep it." That was the same year I played Scrooge. He had a different relationship to money until he learned his purpose was to let it flow.

With formative experiences such as these, I began to believe that I was truly a Child of Good Fortune who was fished out of the millpond and given to a childless couple, my adoptive parents. In the fable, his initiation ultimately takes him to the underworld, where he must pluck three golden hairs from the devil's head. More on that later. Right now we are living with the question, "How will William and Andy cover their medical expenses?" So far the answer is a shiny quarter and an old penny.

My father, once he retired, had a great struggle with alcohol. In a vicious circle, his guilt aggravated his longing for escape. His drinking habit had been incubating for years in a heavy drinking society with martini lunches, a long cocktail hour before dinner, cocktail parties, and too much time alone on the road. The rhythm of going to the office sober on Monday curtailed his weekend binges for a time. When he retired all bets were off. He retired early, at sixty-two—whether at the company's initiative or his own I never knew. Without the constraints of work, he was a hard drinker, more than a fifth of whiskey a day. He would pass out and start again when he woke up. It was a death wish. He would be thumping around in the middle of the night. We were always afraid he would fall down the stairs. His prowling would summon my mother, self-medicated with Vodka herself, to coax him back to his bedroom. The nagging enraged him. He was angry with himself and haunted by the phantom of his domineering father. He was wracked with regret for never fulfilling his promise as an aeronautical engineer, for being passed over by the company, for being stuck in a management job that didn't tap his engineering roots. Mom stuck by him with the stubborn persistence of a Swede and annoyed the hell out of him. I felt powerless to help them climb out of the tragic self-destructive pattern they were in.

Once I came home from prep school for Easter vacation. I think I was a junior. When I saw what shape my parents were in, I flew into a rage. They were drinking away their lives. It was suicidal, no exit. This "Long Day's Journey into Night" psychodrama was too much for me. Nothing I said made a dent. On Saturday night before Easter, I violently swept a bowl of nuts from the table in front of my shocked parents. The nuts scattered across the room, and I stormed from the house.

My anger at my parents' illness spilled over into suicidal thoughts as I stood on the Main Street Bridge and watched the dark flowing waters. Too cold. Too shallow. Pointless. It was all so pointless. I was deeply depressed—Jimmy Stewart just before his angel appears in *It's a Wonderful Life*. I chose life, a cup of coffee, a piece of pie, and a smoke at the greasy spoon refuge. A Hispanic migrant worker came in and bought a six-pack to round out payday. Receiving his change, with a big smile, he pushed it across the counter toward me. Stunned by his generosity, I protested. "I've got money." He said, "Keep it, you look like you need it more than I do."

At the low point of my dark night of the soul this unknown man came, then disappeared into Easter Saturday midnight. Downy flakes of snow began to float peacefully earthward in the still air. The black waters flowing under the bridge, the crisp air, the warmth of compassion behind the gift money changed me. The descent into hell turned to Easter dawn. The tomb opened, and I heard bells. Resurrection! My hard heart opened like a white lily in gratitude toward my parents, forgiveness and hope for them, forgiveness for myself, and renewed belief in spiritual guidance. There was always and would always be a helping hand in time of need.

My number crunching turned up some interesting facts. Ironically, if I died, we, or, rather Andy, would have no financial problem. Grief and loneliness would be problems, but money, small consolation, from my retirement account and insurance would help pay the bills. But I ruled out my dying, based on my intuition/experience that I was to continue for a time in this world to fulfill a task. We had to have Plan A if I were to live an unspecified number of years, which I was elated to have the opportunity to attempt. Plan B (death and an insurance payoff), a very poor second, was the backup.

What would our annual health care costs be if I were to survive more than a year, the short time allotted for those who had the big one, glioblastoma multiforme phase IV? Skip all this if you think this sort of thing will never happen to you or if numbers make you ill. I projected an annual medical expense of about $8,000 not covered by insurance. This would cover co-payments for very expensive medicine ($500 a dose if you're uninsured, until your money runs out and Medicaid kicks in); a long-term health care policy; complementary treatments like Iscador, therapeutic baths, and art therapy; visits to our oncologist and family physician.

Most people I knew were struggling from paycheck to paycheck. We had saved as best we could on a teacher's salary. The burst of the dot-com bubble vaporized the inheritance we had received from Andy's father. This was a bitter pill following the "irrational exuberance" of illusory wealth. We owned our home with little debt and had a modest nest egg in a TIAA-CREF

403(b) account. Our house, owner-built for $50,000 in 1979, was our chief asset. It was also our chief liability, since the tax bite had grown to $6,000 a year. I will spare you a rant. Retirement would be tight. We had medical insurance, God be praised, with a $6,000 deductible and a twenty-percent co-pay. My salary of $40,000 after thirty years of teaching would end in three months. Andy's income would continue. Disability insurance would kick in at $28,000 annually, seventy percent of my former salary. Two months before the outbreak of my illness, I talked Andy into our signing up for a long-term-care insurance policy. Why? We were both healthy and could hardly afford the extra payments, unless of course one of us actually fell seriously ill. Now I'm glad we had signed on. I have my father's conservative mindset to thank.

I knew so little of such things before my illness. A delegation of friends in the Hawthorne Valley Administration came to our house a week after surgery to fill us in. Andy was on paid leave of absence through the Christmas holiday until January 6. To sum up: annual loss of income $12,000 plus discontinuing an annual contribution of $4,000 to a retirement account and increased medical expenses of $8,000 annually for two to three years if I should live so long. That's about $24,000 less per year than we were counting on for "our" retirement—you know, the golden years, cruises, exotic journeys, creative hobbies, etcetera.

Our course was clear. We would spend whatever it took to restore my wounded body to balance. We had $33,000 in investments. We'd use that first, keeping a respectful distance from my retirement account until we had to tap into it for medical emergencies like this.

Cue the miracle. Pennies from heaven rained on the Child of Good Fortune. I won't say who helped. It was a wise and loving couple who together have walked the cancer path. They offered us friendship, guidance, and courage to thread the maze. They wanted to ensure that I had the complementary therapies that I chose. They also wanted to ensure that Andy had discretionary money to allocate as she saw the need. They gave us a very generous GIFT. This gift freed us from the immediate financial anxiety that accompanies such an illness and opened therapeutic opportunities that our habitual thrift would have vetoed. We now could make decisions for healing outside the orthodox allopathic medical box and insurance systems. With an illness this serious, their support was actually a gift of life and hope.

Enter friends. Word had gone out that I was planning a trip to the famous Lucas Cancer Clinic in Arlesheim, Switzerland, for further treatment when my radiation therapy was complete. Within two weeks the money appeared. A brother had delivered the first $1,000 and consulted with me. "Who are your close friends that I could ask on your behalf? These should be people whom you know who want to help, have the ability to help, and are waiting for the go-ahead. With your permission, I will ask them each for a gift for your treatment." Fifteen friends made that commitment. This was no tax write-off; this was pure gift, Star Money. One man said in his note, "If this isn't what money is for, I don't know what is."

Another brother put up $1,000 to cover our tab at the Farm Store. Checks came in Christmas cards along with beautiful expressions of love, hope, and faith that I would come through this trial. A benefit concert for a fellow cancer survivor* and myself was arranged, initiating a complementary therapy fund. We were to be the first beneficiaries. The specter of the Poor House skulked into the shadows. The sun of generosity broke through the clouds. A rainbow bridging from heaven to earth appeared. There actually was a Pot o' Gold at the end of it. Thank you dear friends, thank you *Spirit of Generosity*. We receive and honor your blessing daily with grateful hearts.

> *Take no thought for your life, what ye shall eat, or what ye shall drink; nor yet for your body, what ye shall put on. Is not the life more than meat, and the body more than raiment? Behold the fowls of the air: for they sow not, neither do they reap nor gather into barns; yet your heavenly Father feedeth them. Are ye not much better than they?...*

---

*   We shared our path for some months to come. Our friend crossed the threshold in the spring of 2007.

Consider the lilies of the field, how they grow; they toil not, neither do they spin: And yet I say unto you, that even Solomon in all his glory was not arrayed like one of these." (Matt. 6:25–26, 28–29)

Helpless and ill, I had been arrayed with the rainbow cloak of the love of my friends and community.

FIRE

I HAD ENTERED THE TWILIGHT zone. The weekly work rhythm thirty years in the making had vanished like smoke, along with my former identity as a teacher. Responsibilities, schedules, agendas, deadlines, lesson preparation, correcting student work, committee work, working around the clock and against the clock all flew out the window. Eternity was left: the sky, the trees, the rocks, the stars. The monkey mind stopped chattering. I abided now in spacious emptiness. The wondering, wandering soul experienced in the swaying trees, the whisper of the wind, the rattle of a leaf, the winter sun, and drifting clouds a poignant forgotten beauty that had been buried by pressing commitments, by busyness. *"'Tis a gift to be simple / 'tis a gift to be free / 'tis a gift to come down where we ought to be ...."* was my song. I had been so busy DOING, without looking up, that I had forgotten BEING. I had forgotten BREATHING. My work had been removed. My life had been restored. "Get a life!" Here it was. Here I am.

Otto, our grandchild, one and a half years old at the time of my illness, frequently came visiting. Together we would build a fire. With his tiny hand in mine, we would descend into the mysterious basement. We would do manly work together of gathering kindling and logs, Otto imitating my every gesture with absolute attention. Together we would lift the logs into the canvas tote and cart them up the stairs.

I crumpled paper. He threw it in the fireplace. Then, according to the wisdom of the elders, came the kindling followed by seasoned logs. Promethean Gramps would magically ignite the match of volcanic sulphur and Phosphorus, the light bearer. As the fire blazed up in elemental magnificence, Otto, deep brown eyes ablaze in the reflected glory, would hunker down and point with both arms, his whole body, and his lively soul toward the blaze and NAME it: *FFFFIIIIEEEE!* "FIRE"— alive, alight, hot, dancing, flaming, flickering.

Quest-for-Fire Gramps, the fool on the hill, witnessed day after day Otto's encounter with *fire, wood, water, sun, moon, snow, bird, stone, tree.* The old man heard through Otto's joy the universe of language, of meanings, lighting up as objects-sounds newly minted from the matrix of the worldwide All. This miraculous, explosive acquisition of language was occurring for Otto at Christmas time, the season of the birth of the Holy Child and the rebirth of the light. *"In the beginning was the Word and the Word was with God and the Word was God.... All things were made by him; without him was not anything made that was made. In him was life; and the life was the light of men"* (John 1:1,3).

Gramps was so habituated to his own thought processes that words were worn clichés. But, through Otto's delight in the newness of everything, I could reexperience the birth of the priceless gift of language. The primal Word, fountainhead of meaning, was received and individualized as a spiritual gift in the little man. He also was a Holy Child, like every child, receiving the gift of the Mother tongue, like a golden treasure bestowed by a king. In the beginning, Child-Mother-Father-World are one. Then differentiation begins. At first, "Mama" denotes both mother and father like Adam and Eve before consciousness of their separation into two.

Angels hovered round to learn what names Adam would bestow upon the elements of undivided creation. The sacred names united sound, perception, light, thought, imagination, image, memory, and intense feeling with the gestures and qualities of things. Like Helen Keller first experiencing "water" as word-element-idea, every thing, every word was indelibly precious to Otto. "Dog," "rock," "up," "down," "ball," "red" impressed themselves on his eager senses, mind, and lips. He joyfully grasped things with direct perception-conception-naming and full body participation. There is nothing to explain or define because everything in his expanding universe was self-evident. The name is the thing.

Before my eyes, Otto's vocabulary was growing exponentially, daily, at one and a half years old. Efforts to record this daily proliferation were futile. All the words of all dictionaries were but the dried leaves of once-living experience. All compendia of the sciences, likewise, were but the composting mold of past experience: zoology, biology, etymology, entomology, physiology, psychology, geology, anthropology were all twigs and branches of the Logos, the World Word, the unitary Tree of Life/Tree of Knowledge. Each word, a leaf of this infinitely ramifying tree, had its own unique sound, form, and meaning. The infinite suppleness and refined mobility coordinating larynx, breath, tongue, lips, teeth, and hearing produced such wonders as "ball" which rolls roundly off Otto's tongue. How soft, fresh, flowing was "water." "Rock" was round, hard, solid, and crystalline. "Blue" was cool, mysterious, vast. "Squirrel" skittered and rippled as it rhythmically bounded along the high wire. The fire said "crackle." Watching Otto gaze with such pure attention at the fire before us embodied this truth: "You must become a child to enter the kingdom of heaven."

Someday I could even tell him stories, but for now words were renewing the world.

CHOP WOOD, CARRY WATER, GO TO DOCTOR

WITHOUT CONSULTATION OR CHOICE, my life had drastically been simplified. My sole—or should I say "soul"—focus, was to do whatever it took to stay alive, with Andy at my right hand. Calendar and clock were irrelevant to me. I was off the grid, on solar time by day and star time by night. As I recovered from surgery, hibernating midday naps were precious while the ebb and flow of deep breathing renewed every cell. Now that the post-surgical Decadron had all worn off, I found great contentment watching the flickering flames of the fire.

But there was a flip side: Dealing with the unknown. Two cancer survivors had told me independently, "You have to be actively engaged in your recovery." "You must be your own advocate." "The men in the white coats will give conflicting opinions. You have to make the decisions. It's your body." Another friend told me forcefully, *"Heal yourself!"* That command, rang in the air. And the wise Doctor Incao observed, "Your ego involvement with your illness provides the healing force to overcome it. A person can eat any number of carrots, for example, as a special cancer diet, but it is the ego resolve to do it that is the agent of healing, not the carrots."

Sitting peacefully by the fireside was part, but only part, of the equation. I, or rather we, had to roll up our sleeves to engage the illness on all fronts. What were the roots of the cancer? What must I transform in myself so the cancer would not recur? What were the sustaining therapies that might cheat death? In the time left to me, what might I do to serve the Children of the Future I had glimpsed in vision? If I were to continue to live for only a year or a year and a half, how should I use my time? Who could I confide in that would take seriously the experience of the *Spirit of Generosity?* How could I share the insights I had received about the nature of the child—the power of the will, the power of compassion, the power of imagination— without it being reduced to mere words?

So a pendulum swung in my soul between contemplative feelings of peace, contentment, and the precious joy of life, and on the other pole, urgency of purpose, arrangements for the future, strategies for survival, internet research, and an endless round of medical appointments. Half my waking hours would be spent ferrying between appointments. The WAITING ROOM became a second home. As the *I Ching*, the ancient Chinese book of wisdom, observes: "Waiting is."

In less than two weeks after my surgery, my appointment calendar for December quickly filled. Radiation therapy began in the middle of the month at the Cavel Cancer Treatment Center in nearby Hudson, New York. A preliminary MRI was given, the first since surgery, and X-rays taken to map the area for treatment. Lead alloy molds were made to shield the rest of the brain from radiation, targeting only the surgical site and surrounding tissue of the left parietal-occipital lobe. A plastic net was molded to my face; this net was clamped to the radiation table to hold my head in a fixed position during radiation. This narrow bed was rolled on a fixed track into a position exactly determined by intersecting laser beams. The particle accelerator streamed the prescribed radiation in units called *Grays* (for Dr. Gray, not gray matter) at precise angles to the site from which the tumor was removed. There was a little buzzing sound, a short burst of the prescribed dosage. The massive metallic arm that projected what I fondly call the Death Ray rotated electronically into position to irradiate the same site from the opposite side. After the first planning, scanning, and targeting visit, the whole procedure took only fifteen minutes each time. There was little waiting around. The technicians were cheerful, considerate, and communicative, knowing that for some patients having their head clamped to a table is somewhat out of the comfort zone. It all had a sci-fi vibe for me. So what if I should lose my hair as a side effect of treatment. That hadn't happened yet and, when it did, I would be skinhead cool.

Thirty-three doses of the radiation therapy were prescribed. Thirty-three is a lifetime maximum dosage. Coincidentally, in my highly charged universe of signs and symbols, it was also the number of years of Christ's life. I immediately appreciated Dr. Kim, the radiologist. He was completely frank in responding to our many questions. Like a nightmare or a movie with a psychopathic killer or lethally programmed android, this particular cancer in the majority of cases refuses to die. The Terminator has to bring out the heavy-duty artillery to keep the beast down. Like uprooting an aphid-infested plant, one soon realizes that all the tenacious root hairs remain in the pot or cranium as the case may be.

Any one of the cells can reseed (the opposite of recede) the whole process. I say nuke 'em.

Andy was my chauffeur at first. A cadre of close friends signed on round robin to ferry me to the six weeks of radiation treatment. In addition, Andy and I both had the oil dispersion baths once a week. We each had a gift certificate for Rosen massage therapy given by close family friends who knew its benefits. We also had a December appointment with Dr. Susan Weaver, our oncologist, and an appointment with Dr. Margaretha Hertle, our family physician who prescribed the complementary therapies and remedies that would support the healing process, including the weekly infusion of Iscador. Andy also had two trips to the chiropractor scheduled for herself. Being this sick, though I felt fine, was a full-time job. So far that is twenty-nine appointments in a month and a half, plus a trip to the mechanic. There was time off for Christmas and New Year's. We were hitting this illness with everything we had.

In addition to this demanding regimen, once a week I would walk to a near neighbor's house for music therapy. Gili Lev is a Juilliard-trained pianist who plays at school festivals, gives local concerts, and supports concerts benefiting the school's music program. Gili was also a parent of a precocious child in my class, Shai, who is certainly one of the Children of Future, ready and willing to share her own musical gift. Gili played Bach and Mozart for me; just the four of us were there: Bach, Mozart, Gili, and I. With eyes closed and heart and soul wide open, the sublime musical architecture raised me up to realms of reverence and praise never known before. What could heal me if not such music? If it was too late for my body to be healed, it was not for my soul. Having made the ascent up Bach's fugue ladder, now airborne, Mozart's heavenly playfulness would ripple through my body, resonating through and around my bones and lungs and heart and larynx in the aerated pulse of blood and through the water-dance of my cells. My God! Life forces of great joy bubbled from this inexhaustible fountain of youth. Scintillating synapses were launching fireworks worthy of Bilbo Baggins's birthday. Lifted on wings of melody, forgetting self, I was privileged to ride this undulating magic carpet through auroras of dawn to celestial climes.

When the music stopped, I would wipe my tears away and we would have tea and nuts and dried berries and talk about the children and what my doctors thought. No, I was not going to die. Not with this kind of medicine. Side effects may cause ecstatic states, dancing, prayer, praise to Glory, and permanent lift-off. Take only as prescribed. Thank you Gili, Johann, and Wolfgang. Thank you, Lord, for the rejuvenating force of music! This sweet, swinging singing celestial sphere is the spiritual home of the Children of the Future.

After daily appointments, I would come back to the nest, the sanctuary, to eat and nap. In the afternoon I would split some kindling, haul up some logs and keep the home fire burning. The seasoned wood released the stored-up sunlight, *Sol Invictus*, against winter's cold and dark. God willing, the hearth fire would not go out.

When darkness fell, there would come a knock at the door. The Food Chain! What delectable home-cooked meal would we be having tonight? In would come a family from my class. There were enough of them to take us into January. We would chat for an hour by the fire about all manner of things. I was so glad to see again this karmic cast of characters and their loving families. I knew I could no longer be their teacher, but the longing was still there from my side and theirs. I hauled out from Ward's Hoard ancient artifacts that would interest my students: a Civil War revolver and saber and a copper-headed tomahawk. Whatever shadows of deep concern lurked in the background did not surface in the good cheer and affection that warmed the room. Friends and the children could see that I was doing well and was in very good spirits, the Scrooge Rebirth Effect. Though I was incommunicado, separated from my community except for homeopathic doses of the Food Chain, reports would go forth on the grapevine that William was doing well.

So we headed toward Christmas and the birth of the Holy Child. Words of Angelus Silesius given me by Andy fifteen years before came resoundingly back: "I must become like Mary / and bring forth Christ in me, if I would be blessed / for all eternity."

COCOON

W<small>E HUNKERED DOWN OVER</small> Christmas. I was housebound except for medical excursions. The stimulus of a shopping trip to the mall would have been suicidal. We tried to keep it simple and inward. Christmas cards and wishes came down like snowflakes. All those caring people who constellated what I had glimpsed as the Medicine Wheel still knew little of my condition. It was time for a community letter. The following missive was available at the check out register at the Hawthorne Valley Farm Store.

WARD EMERGES FROM COCOON!

Epiphany 2006
Dear Friends,

Blessings on your New Year!

Thank you for all your healing prayers and friendship. Your good thoughts on my behalf have sent a stream of light and love toward me from all points of the compass. Andy and I are grateful beyond words to be sustained in this way by our community of friends and neighbors. This prayer circle has been especially powerful through the holy nights of Hanukkah and Christmas....

Imagine you are me opening a Christmas card. There have been many cards. One sees good wishes written there of *light, joy, peace,* and *love.* Only now the simple words spring to life with a clear experience of the warm friendship of the sender. Now imagine that you go to sleep at night, breathing peacefully like a child. Your dreams ring with a great celestial choir of all the people you know with their angels behind them, encircling this sleeping child (you-me). They are singing a celestial lullaby of love and peace on earth. The child wakes up in the morning feeling completely refreshed and grateful for the new day. All that energy has gone right into the child. The songs of the night fade away, but the miracle of day holds its own revelations seen in the light of the night's voyage. Thank you.

❧

Now, down to earth. Rarely in our small circles has an illness been so public without the benefit of media coverage. We are grateful for the blanket of privacy you have provided. But I am about to make my first visit to the Farm Store, and we need to scope this out together so it's possible to buy some vegetables without creating gridlock. So, I am writing this open letter to communicate the current state of my nation to all of you who have taken such an active interest in my well-being. My hope is that I can address Frequently Asked Questions all at once, rather than sequentially. Such as: HOW IS WILLIAM DOING?

Chronology: Headaches and mental fogginess in early November. Loss of typing skills, trouble teaching. MRI at recommendation of Dr. Steven Kaufman. Brain tumor discovered. November 10: Albany Medical Center MRI's and full body CT scan. Brain surgery scheduled for November 17! (Stuart Summer substitutes in the fourth grade followed by Candace Christiansen). Three days of observation and intravenous Dilantin (anti-seizure medicine) at Albany Med. Branko Furst, our friend and a highly respected anesthesiologist, escorts us through the labyrinth to pre-op. He stays with Andy, Claire, Rosie, and Billy during much of the morning. Josh is at home looking after Otto. Stella Elliston arrives for moral support. Dr. German and Dr. Friedlich (Dr. "Peaceful," who could ask for a better team?) perform surgery on left parietal-occipital lobe and remove a plum-sized mass of tumor in two and a half hours. Branko appears like an angel to William and says, "It's over." William spends two and a half days in the hospital and is taken back to hearth and home.

Excarnation: The patient has had a major out-of-body visionary experience, which may be summed up by the ancient phrase "Die and become." (He is now restored to apparent normality with wisps of the vision remaining). The patient is overjoyed to be home! He talks a lot and cannot sleep for two and a half weeks as he is gradually weaned off powerful doses of an anti-inflammatory drug called Decadron (a steroid). Laboratory analysis confirms the tumor was an aggressive (fast growing) glioblastoma multiforme. Not a good thing.

Landing: The Wards' steep learning curve has begun. Andy is given a leave of absence from her work in the kindergarten (at the busiest season of the year) to support William (thank God for nurse Andy!). A week before Christmas vacation, William meets with the Council and resigns from class teaching (1976–2005) to devote himself to the next chapter in his life, where each day is a gift, not a rewarding (pun intended) duty. The Wards cope with a flood of research, good wishes, bills, appointments, future tripping, calls, unknowns, and therapeutic options from their command post on Old Wagon Road. Thank God for the Food Chain! (Symptomatic of my current condition is a noticeable shift toward greater gratitude, invoking heavenly help, and the more frequent use of exclamation points!)

Prognosis: I am in God's hands. On the earthly plane Andy and I are pursuing every available therapy. Statistically, only twenty percent of the people with this form of cancer have a life expectancy exceeding two years. Some exceed seven years and have articles written about them. I intend to join the latter category, if not set a new benchmark for longevity at the far end. Louis, one of my caregivers in the hospital said to me, "If the Lord says, 'Come, Louis,' I go." He also said, "You are not going anywhere. It is not your time. You have work to do." That is what I think, too.

Treatment: In consultation with Dr. Margaretha Hertle; Dr. Weaver, a neuro-oncologist associated with Albany Medical Center; and Dr. Kim, a radiologist affiliated with the Cavel Cancer Center in Hudson we are pursuing a therapeutic regimen that includes standard allopathic treatment for this disease and a spectrum of complementary treatments and medicines.

Radiation: The radiation therapy involves daily trips to Hudson five days per week for thirty-three consecutive doses of radiation targeting the area of my brain from which most of the tumor was removed. If you notice loss of my brain function try not to let it show. If you think my brain is functioning about the median level of absurdity or is actually more lucid, feel free to give me positive feedback. I am extremely grateful that the tumor was accessible and could be removed without affecting the centers of speech and movement. I can imagine myself restricted in movement, but not talking...!

Chemotherapy: I also am taking Temodar chemotherapy, 160 milligrams per day during radiation treatment, which is designed to interfere with reproduction of the hyperactive cancer cells. Temodar became standard treatment for this type of brain cancer in conjunction with radiation therapy about three years ago based on Danish studies. When the radiation ends, Temodar dosage will increase to 400 milligrams daily for five days, followed by twenty-three days off in a monthly rhythm for a year. Thank God (there I go again) for health insurance, for without it our house would be on the market and we would be living in our igloo or car. The medicine alone is $500 per day. It is not making me nauseous, but it would if I were picking up the whole tab.

As grateful as I am for the advances in allopathic medicine, the doctors we have consulted have a coldly scientific, statistical view of this illness, scripted not to get one's hopes up. The patient is urged to enjoy life (while one can...which is exactly what I am doing). This is where alternative, complementary therapies come in.

Anthroposophically Extended Medicine: Under the guidance of Dr. Hertle, I have been treated with Iscador, a mistletoe extract, which is a powerful stimulant to the immune system. This treatment, developed by Rudolf Steiner and Dr. Ita Wegman, has about eighty years of medical use behind it for a variety of illnesses. It is widely known in Europe where they have more experience with its healing properties. Here it is less known with the exception of a few research hospitals, which are studying its benefits. This is a remarkable medicine that I cannot recommend highly enough.

Additionally, I am receiving weekly *oil dispersion baths*. This is a powerful alternative therapy used for years with great success in Camphill and abroad. I highly recommend you look into this if you feel the therapeutic need, as I do, to make a change in your life in body, soul, and spirit.

Complementary Therapies: I have visited a remarkable man in New York City who has devoted his life to healing. His name is Zeev Kolman. His *bioenergetic* approach to grave illness is a great contrast to allopathic medicine's paradigm. "I feel the power." That is all I'll say about it right now....

We have benefited from the healing hands of Lee Cheek, a *Rosen Method Bodywork* practitioner in South Egremont. And Corey Schifano, a dear friend, paid a massage house call. Nicole Furnee has given many rhythmic massage sessions for my feet. We have offers of help from professional acupuncturists, who also can give guidance for powerful herbal remedies derived from Chinese medicine. Without mentioning more names, I want to include in the therapeutic circle looking after us: macrobiotic chefs, a painting therapist, therapeutic eurythmy, music therapy, *Journey* work, a Christian Community priest, the Food Chain, and dear old friends.

Clinic: In early March I intend to travel to Arlesheim, Switzerland, for a two-week stay at the Lucas Clinic followed by a two-week stay at Casa di Cura di Andrea Christoforo overlooking Lago Maggiore. I'm halfway there already. Their therapeutic regimen rivals what we can find here in our own amazing backyard! I look forward to this retreat.

Finances: Rachel Schneider has been a bulwark of support by offering insurance/organizing/bill paying guidance as we wind our way through the labyrinthine paperwork of our medical situation.

A joint benefit is being arranged for a fellow cancer patient and myself to help defray clinic costs. This initiative is consciously intended to launch an ongoing fund for people with similar needs outside the mainstream forms of medical insurance.

We have also received substantial financial backup from personal friends who want to guarantee that we have the funds necessary to choose appropriate therapies as needed. Another friend has set up a tab at the Farm Store for us.

The *Spirit of Generosity* is alive and well! So is the *Spirit of Gratitude*!

The Fourth Grade: I am delighted to report that the school has found an excellent teacher for the fourth grade class, my friend Theo Lundin. Not only has he biked across the country; not only has he taken a class through eight grades at the Mountain Laurel School in New Paltz, New York; not only does he have a wonderful wife (Twana); but he is also cheerful, positive, and a dedicated Waldorf teacher, willing to offer a helping hand in time of need. I've known Theo for ten years and couldn't be more confident knowing that he is now responsible for this remarkable class of amazing individuals in the fourth grade.

In conclusion, let me come full circle: We have been lifted up by your kindness and prayers. Now you know as much of the story as I can put to paper. I will emerge from my cocoon and visit with old friends at the Farm Store in the near future.

Love,
William

P.S. The Surgeon General warns: William is subject to sei-zures (i.e., quite unexpectedly he might seize you in a bear hug without provocation). As my daughter Rosie warned her peers at the threshold of a visit to me, "Get ready for some lovin'."

I did emerge from my seclusion, as the letter to the community forewarned, early in the New Year, right at Epiphany. My forays to the Farm Store did cause gridlock. I could see the headlines: CAN-CER ROCK STAR TRAGICALLY SMOTHERED BY WELL WISHERS. The choice was either to embrace old friends and well wishers, engage in updating them with assurances of my progress and descriptions of my therapies, and receive helpful advice from their experience; or put on a ski mask to try to get the groceries. Andy would also get stuck in the store responding to the blessings, questions, and suggestions of friends. Sometimes Claire would bring us our gro-ceries; or Josh, our son-in-law, who was working at the Farm Store, could bag a few items for us for a stealth pickup. But we didn't need much. The Food Chain was still going, and our Farm Store tab was covered by our generous friends.

EPIPHANY

SOLSTICE, HANUKKAH, CHRISTMAS, THE Holy Nights, and New Year's were especially poignant and profound. The simple light-ing of the dinner candles and saying a blessing on the meal had an eternal, ritual quality celebrating life and light enhanced, not diminished, by the specter of cancer. A daily prayer as we blessed our food was, "Keep us mindful of the Children of the Future." All these festivals, connected with the solar year, celebrated the rebirth of the light from winter's night. I felt the resurgence of sun forces countering the side effects of fatigue from radiation and chemo. Perhaps I would come through the eye of the needle. Perhaps I would gain a new balance that would keep recurrence of the cancer at bay.

From our breakfast table we would see the morning sunrise. The blue ridge line of the eastern hills seen from our window marked the limits of the sun's farthest journey to the south where it "stood still" (sol-stice) and rose at the same place for three consecutive days following December 21. From then on sunrise would come a little earlier each day as the sun moved north toward the notch in the ridge. I too was coming back to the light.

January 6 is celebrated as Three Kings day, the coming of the Magi from the East, whose star wisdom had prophesied the birth of the Holy Child. They found him in Bethlehem and offered their gifts of gold, frankincense, and myrrh. This was an epiphany — the appearance of the divine as the Christ Child. It is celebrated on the same day as the baptism of Christ by John. I read these accounts with the deepest interest, seeking a path toward the rebirth of the Holy Child in myself. Against the cosmic backdrop of the festivals of the year the many gifts I was already receiving became abundantly clear: family, love, light, life, healing.

There were counter-forces weighing on the other side of the scale: isolation, doubt, fear, darkness, and illness; but I felt the balance tipping toward rebirth. The image of emerging from a cocoon was especially resonant for me. In my condition, the pattern of entombment and emergence recurred with stunning regularity. Coming out of the tubular sarcophagus of the MRIs was always such a moment. Coming out from the daily radiation lock down was similar. Waking up with the sun to each new day from the cocoon of sleep carried the same joyous message.

Likewise there was the nightly journey of the soul and spirit (*astral body* and "*I*") to the starry realms while the *physical* and *etheric* bodies were refreshed in the bliss of deep sleep. The oil dispersion baths were another cocooning-rebirth process of transformation. What a paradox it was that immobilizing the body, tightly swaddling it in darkness, allowed the soul forces to become mobile and active, stimulated by the plant essence permeating the bath. Osiris's entombment in the floating casket, his envelopment in the tree, and subsequent rescue mythologically repeats the theme of initiatory death that leads to crossing the threshold between this world and the spiritual world. In the New Testament, Lazarus also experiences this rebirth process and is born to new life. The death, entombment, and resurrection of Christ raises this archetype of rebirth to the cosmic level.

Strange that I had to be physically bound in the winding sheets of the baths to free up my soul space. Otherwise, life was just a bunch of running around chasing thought formations that seemed important at the time. But where is the time to dwell in silence, in inwardness of soul, until the essence of one's being grows wings to fly?

The first time I saw the MRI scans, I was shocked to see several of the horizontal cross sections reveal with absolute clarity the form of a butterfly at the center of the brain, entombed at Golgotha, the place of the skull. This was another epiphany. Roll back the stone. Set it free.

I thought of my mother frequently in the cocoon hour of the oil baths. She too had been bound by illness and set free. She died July 2, 1994, at age eighty-eight. This was a great release from the prison of her failing body. As we were burying Mom's body on a sunny day a few days later, a monarch butterfly fluttered by. I had written a poem to her the day before, written as though she were speaking. The poem included a butterfly. Now it was flying by. From that point on, tuned to the butterfly emblem of life emerging from death, the psyche from the body, I began seeing monarchs with surprising frequency. I wondered if I always thought of Mom when one appeared, or did one appear as her messenger whenever I tuned to Mom? No matter. I could simply observe, withhold judgment and enjoy the synchronicity of inexplicable, meaningful coincidence written on butterfly wings.

OUTSIDE

I love these yellow roses,
Just like my wedding day,
But now we've talked long enough,
I've nothing more to say;
I've finished all my tasks,
I've paid all my bills,
What more can I ask
Than what the spirit wills.

The lock's worn out,
I have no doubt
Nothing holds me here,
Confined no more,
An open door,
And the way is clear.

The best time for sunning
Is in the dawn's early rays
While the birds are singing
Their morning song of praise.

You need not hold my hand,
My journey has begun,
I have the strength to stand
And go out in the sun.

How light I feel today,
And I slept so well,
Where will I go, you wish to know,
It's hard for me to tell...
But would it be a wonder,
If I were a seed,
For light to raise me sunward
As flowering, fruitful tree?
I accept this mystery,

The chrysalis transformed,
Sets the homebound monarch free
To bright day reborn.

So now, by grace, the spirit's art,
The door springs open wide,
And day-clear light fills my heart
As I step outside.

At exactly the same moment, my brother and I had arrived back home for the funeral, from Pennsylvania and New York respectively. Dave had the key to open the door, the door that Mom always kept locked. Like the grandfather's clock that "stopped short, never to go again when the old man died," the locking mechanism spontaneously sprang apart in his hand as Andy and I looked on in wonder.

As a cancer patient I am still in the tomb-womb-cocoon stage as pupa and pupil. But I experience the transformation of the monarch butterfly in its jeweled coffin as a real picture—not a poetic metaphor—of the soul's metamorphosis. Such a true Imagination is a gift of hope, eloquent evidence of benevolence and grace for all facing the open door to the next world. As a humble chrysalis in crisis, I place my life in Christ's hands. He knocks on the jeweled coffin and the Monarch, the Self, is set free.

HANDS OF HEALING

DEAR FRIEND AND NEIGHBOR Gili Lev called me one morning, wondering whether I would accompany her to a famous healer she had heard about—Zeev Kolman. Gili, whose daughter Shai had been in my class for three years, was the musician who played Bach's *Goldberg Variations* for me weekly as an

integral part of my healing process. Two of her friends, both
of whom I happened to know, had been to Zeev and came back
with glowing reports. One friend had had breast cancer, which
went into remission after her visits. The other had suffered from
debilitating colitis for nearly two years. After a handful of visits
with Zeev, she was back on her feet and full of life, the way I
remembered her.

These two women didn't know one another, but had both been
steered toward this mysterious healer independently and told Gili
about their experiences. Would I be interested?!?!

I had been given about ten books about cancer. I had been
given another ten inspirational tapes. I couldn't find the soul space
to receive all the inspiration and advice that was coming my way,
but what Zeev offered was not words. Healing power streamed
through his hands. Worth looking into.

Gili and I took the commuter train from Hudson down to Penn
Station and walked uptown to Zeev's office on West 57th Street.
The Big Apple, Fun City, I Love NY. Out of the cocoon and onto
the streets. WOW! Gili had gone to Juilliard for her musical training. I had gone to Columbia in the late sixties. She led the way as I,
the country boy with cancer, gazed at the tall buildings. Gili kept
me from getting hit by cabs en route to my healing session, as I
coped with the hyper-stimulation of the big city.

Laughter, black humor, delight in the absurd were vital to
my recovery. Nothing debilitates one's sense of humor like a life-
threatening tumor. A friend told me this one on the way to a blood
test. I usually don't remember jokes, but this one stuck.

There was this minister. He died and went to heaven. St. Peter
greeted him and gave him a monk's robe, sandals, and a belt and
led him to a simple cabin in the beautiful forest of the ministers'
section of Paradise. The cabin had a warm fire, contemplative
solitude, books, and everything he needed for his comfort. One
day there was a great commotion at the gates. Thinking it must
be someone important, the minister looked out and saw a New
York City cabdriver being given a hero's welcome. He was arrayed
in a colorfully embroidered robe and golden sandals, and given
a scepter and a jeweled belt. He was led to a palace with a staff

of servants and a banquet all prepared. The minister felt short-changed. He asked St. Peter why this cabby was being treated so royally, while he, on the other hand, had devoted his entire life to God and received only a simple cabin. St. Peter replied, "While you were preaching, your congregation was bored stiff, thinking of a million other things, or falling asleep. But this cabby's passengers were praying fervently to God for the salvation of their souls."

It must be acknowledged at this point that the Marx Brothers changed medical history when Norman Cousins broke through the solemnity barrier, revealing the hugely therapeutic value of humor in the treatment of illness and pain. "It hurts only when I laugh" is more accurately rendered, "It hurts only when I don't laugh." It all has to do with endorphins and dopamine whose very name begs for a punch line like: What did the drug dealer say to the neutraphil? "Any dope of yours is a dopamine."

I was thrilled to be having such a big-city adventure, since I had hardly been out of my house for two months except for blood tests and doctors' appointments. Here, I saw more people in half an hour on the streets than I did in a year in Columbia County. Their stories streamed by me in endless and eloquent succession, engraved in their expressions and in their funny walking. I felt like a brother from another planet, an illegal alien anthropologist come to observe life on earth, ready to have my solar batteries recharged by the mysterious Zeev Kolman, who operates off the grid in a paranormal universe.

It was damn cold in February, but it didn't matter. It was so exhilarating to be there. We found the building and took the elevator up. Shelley, the receptionist, has a beautiful accent, from the islands (not Long Island or Staten Island), somewhere warm and sultry. She took our pictures and signed us in. I learned later that Zeev could tune himself to one's condition and location just by looking at your picture. In fact you could arrange for a time for Zeev to "visit you" for a healing session without having to come down to the office. That sounds like a good gig, cutting back on transportation overhead, by simply using the astral plane. I would keep an open mind. Beggars can't be choosers.

A broad expanse of wall was covered with pictures of Zeev's former patients. Almost all of them were smiling. Some of the pictures showed Zeev with a client, a bride, a family, a prince, an actress, a shaman, a group of physicians, a beaming child, receiving a medal, hob-knobbing with the wealthy, or waving from the Dead Sea. I begin to think of this smiling man as Zelig, who, chameleon-like, is welcome anywhere to share his healing powers and blessing. As I read inscriptions from celebrities I recognized, most expressed similar sentiments: "Dear Zeev, Thank you for saving my life!" Or "Dear Zeev, Your healing hands are a miracle!"

We sat in the small but comfortable waiting room and sized up the clientele, wondering whether *gullible* is in their dictionary. Who comes to see this man, and how do you find out about him? Scrapbooks of clippings were on the coffee table, articles from magazines, workshop promotionals, testimonial letters of profound gratitude. Hey, maybe I wouldn't need any more radiation by the time Zeev was done with me. There was also a short video on Israel (Zeev is Israeli), and a video of glowing or tearful interviews with former patients. I didn't doubt they were genuine, but I wondered how did he keep his feet on the ground in the midst of so much gratitude. Was there danger of ego inflation? Over the desk there were a hundred copies of a book about him by Hans Holzer, Ph.D., and a salve or ointment for sale—I mean for healing. I was on my guard. My bogusity meter was vibrating violently. But I truly wanted Zeev to be the real deal, since my mainline encouragers were less than enthusiastic about my chances.

On the walls were some paintings by Zeev of three large-eyed figures gazing out from the clouds. This theme was repeated. There was another color photograph of just Zeev's hands with various colors and currents implied. Is it a Kirlian photograph? Whatever that may be. The door opened. Zeev appeared, having just completed a session with a middle-aged woman who was all smiles. He was in his early sixties, about five feet ten inches, strong looking, a brick, salt of the earth. He was energetically (no pun intended) outgoing. He immediately began cracking jokes, speaking in Hebrew to Gili or intermittent English with a thick Israeli accent. His handshake was warm. Was I expecting a joy buzzer? Nothing. His face was weather-beaten and tanned. There was a friendly, warm twinkle in his eye. He paused long enough to consume some cold Chinese food, standing, while Shelley filled him in on appointments. He took Gili first. Periodic laughter wafted through the muffled door, then silence.

Gili came out half an hour later, all smiles. "You're going to enjoy this." Zeev again shook my hand and offered me a chair. His desk was cluttered with mementos. There was also stuff, maybe files, peeking out from beneath it. Feng Shui was not a priority. I glanced at two more walls covered with photographs of more smiling patients and assorted relatives. There was a massage table along one wall. He asked me to tell him about myself and my condition. He listened with great interest. Then he said abruptly, "I have been looking at the colors and layers of your aura. I see where you need help, here, here, and here. Take off your sweater and shirt and lie down." He rolled out the paper bed liner and switched on *Pachelbel's Canon*.

I was not prepared for what came next. Zeev turned on the juice. Holding his hands about a foot above my body, sometimes zeroing in closer, streaming energy rippled over the surface of my skin. I hadn't realized that the surging, rippling, tickling, caressing, thrilling energy would be this palpable, undeniable, and strong! I had expected something more subtle and ethereal. My defenses, objections, skepticism, and determination not to buy any snake oil were evaporating into warmth and wonder. "I'm talking about Good Vibrations, I'm picking up excitations." OK, so where's the battery pack? Plugged into his heel perhaps. Nothing up his sleeve. Am I hearing or only imagining the soft crackle of electricity? My impression is of one of those Sharper Image novelties where a multicolored miniature lightning storm inside a globe responds to touch, like it's alive.

Zeev is speaking softly. "I am cleansing your body of all cancer cells. You are free of cancer. Your body is filled with light. You feel very relaxed and healthy all through your body." Meanwhile, he was moving his hands over what I imagined to be energy channels, chakras, and the 130 centers which he "sees." He placed his hands on either side of my head and a stream of warmth poured in, like a heating pad without the pad. Then back to the full-body cleansing and recharging. It felt halfway between a soft feather brush and rippling electrical water.

"Clench your hands. Now relax them, releasing all tension. Clench your legs. Now let go, all the way down to your toes. Relax the muscles of your face, smooth the muscles of your forehead, breathe easily and deeply from your toes to the top of your head. Release all tension from your body. Let your eyeballs rest in their sockets. Imagine you are in an elevator and the top floor is your head. It is totally at peace, filled with light and health. The elevator descends to the throat...the heart...the solar plexus." The palpable energy is subsiding. By the time the chakra elevator hit the ground floor, the session was over. "How do you feel?" "Wonderful, energized, full of life, all tingly." "Look at yourself in the mirror." I turned around and looked and saw my face with a big wide grin.

Zeev cracked a few more jokes. I realized he was part sage rabbi, part Dr. Feel Good, part stand-up vaudeville comedian. He spoke to Gili in Hebrew, nodding toward me. She explained he wanted to work with me again in about an hour if we could arrange it. He was only half done.

Gili and I compared notes over soup around the corner. "What was that?!" "Who is that guy?" She had browsed the clippings and purchased a book about Zeev to learn more. "What do you think?" Gili asked. "I don't know what to think. My protective shell of skepticism has dissolved. At first I was looking for a cordless battery pack of some kind. Later I thought, Maybe I am in the hands of a hypnotist. This can't be real. We have laws in the physical universe. He can't do this, can he? What's going on?"

Whatever it was, I got another dose of it that afternoon. This time my preconceptions, judgments, and resistance had already been released. I was much more open and present for the treatment. Just lay it on, it feels so good. Same procedure on the surface of things, nearly the same words for the "elevator ride" through the *chakras*. "I am ridding your body of all cancer. You are clean, you feel light and free, you are happy, your head is filled with light." If this is the positive envisioning the inspirational tapes are promoting, bring it on. He says these things with such conviction, rooted in his thirty years' experience with thousands of patients. The healing is not only streaming through his hands but certainly comes through these affirmations also.

At the end of the session, like shaking water off his hands, Zeev forcefully shakes the energy away. "How do you feel? "Wonderful, energized, full of life." He is smiling broadly. "Look at yourself in the mirror. You look younger. There is more color in your cheeks. When you came in you looked like this (imitating a sad, tired face). Now look at yourself. You are ready to go dancing."

This appointment was Martin Luther King day. "I have been to the mountain top... I have seen the promised land... I have seen the glory of the coming of the Lord." "Free at last, free at last, great God Almighty, I am free at last." Was it possible that Zeev's power had indeed cleansed me of cancer as he asserted? Would I be compelled to abandon healthy skepticism about miraculous loopholes in the presumed "laws of nature"? I was hedging my bets. I would continue to see Zeev and continue, obviously, radiation therapy and Temodar chemotherapy. That was a no-brainer, if you'll pardon the expression. Why be exclusive? Seeing Zeev was sooo different from talking with Dr. Weaver, my oncologist. I visualized all my therapists and nurses, ministering to the patient, all smiling, encouraging, all working together. What a team. I could actually get well. I wonder what Dr. Weaver would think of Zeev. Maybe I'll just keep these little visits under my hat.

On subsequent visits to Zeev (about five in all) I grew to appreciate him more and more. He was a Mensch. He knew how to put people at ease and make them laugh. He was encouraging and positive. If he could not help people, he would tell them so. In some cases he would make positive predictions, in others he would refrain. I quickly had gotten over my feeling that there was too much self-promotion in all these pictures on the wall. It was like a family album of Zeev's "children," a karmic tribe of those helped by this unusually gifted man. Like a kindly grandfather, he was proud and pleased of this extended family and had a story about each one. He was a busy man. He saw patients from 9:00 a.m. to 6:00 p.m. He would then take a break and start his evening rounds—all appointments at a distance, often not stopping until midnight. I had to try this out. I talked to the receptionist, who said he preferred to have a session in person, but he had many clients who were perfectly content to have this *bioenergetic healing* without Zeev physically present. Some of them felt his presence at the appointed time, some saw "him" working on them in this non-physical way. I asked Zeev how he does this. He said, "I don't know, but some people say they have seen me with them.... Isn't the universe wonderful?" So with an open mind and an open heart, I took the plunge. I put my credit card down and made an appointment. What did I have to lose?

"You charged an appointment with someone you couldn't see!? You idiot! You are terminally stupid. Call the men in white coats. How do we know Zeev does anything at all during your appoint-ment? He might be seeing a Broadway show on your dime. Is this guy a tax-deductible medical expense? You need your head exam-ined. Evidently they took out the wrong part of your brain."

Unperturbed, I cheerfully respond in my interior dialogue, "Nothing ventured, nothing gained, O ye of little faith."

"Oh, the faith racket. I get it now, you think Zeev is an Oral Roberts wannabee, like those 'Heal!' slaps on the forehead and ecstatic swoons that used to regale you on the day of rest right after the Adventures of Flash Gordon."

"My understanding of the scientific method is to make the experiment and see what happens."

"It's your money. Rather, it was your money, until you threw it away."

"Actually, it never was my money. It is a GIFT from the *Spirit of Generosity* who has guided me to engage my illness and dis-cover what works for me."

I set up another appointment for a week later. I requested it for 11:00 p.m. (Zeev works long hours) so I would be asleep. I speculated that in deep sleep I would receive maximum benefit from these healing forces unhindered by curiosity, skepticism, fear, and the squirrel cage of random thoughts. Unfortunately, I woke up at 10:45 to take a pee.

With fifteen minutes to go, I did my best to relax with my lovely deep breathing. But there was an entirely different mood to anticipating this rendezvous while I was awake. To be honest, I had to consciously work against being spooked at having invited a revenant or projected consciousness of this kindly man to my bedroom in the middle of the night. If he started cracking jokes, it would wake Andy. At exactly 11:00, a strong sensation of warmth streamed into my head and through my arms. The power surge lasted only a few minutes at that level of perceptibility. The tingling, vivifying feeling that I also felt was less dramatic than during the office sessions, but nonetheless perceptible. What could I do but marvel? Zeev gave me hope that extraordinary help was being sent my way, along with the Medicine Wheel, the vision of the Children of the Future, the healing baths, and the personal engagement of my doctors and therapists. I was being treated like that cabbie who went to heaven. Oh, no, had I simply left my heating pad on? No, I had not. I know what I felt. Emerson again: "Spirit is that which is its own evidence."

On a subsequent office visit, as I emerged all smiles, Zeev pointed to a picture on his desk of a handsome twelve-year-old of East Indian extraction. "This boy had the same thing you had. They brought him to me. A month later his tumor was gone. The doctors could find nothing. They were mystified. What else could they conclude, but it had been misdiagnosed. The vanished tumor must not have been there in the first place." He smiled and shrugged. Zeev and I knew better.

JERUSALEM

OLD FRIENDS BEGAN APPEARING in my life again. The grapevine of connectedness was pulsing. Each encounter could be renewal of friendship or farewell. Who knew? But appreciation for one another was deeper than ever under the auspices of cancer. It's ironic that it takes something as dramatic as a brain tumor to rouse the sleeping bonds of friendship. Could we dispense with getting whopped upside the head in order to reinstate social graces in our lives? Whatever happened to hanging out at cafés and shooting the breeze? A bygone era. But cancer was putting on the brakes. Now there was time to just talk and listen and break bread together. There was time to fondly rediscover or recognize for the first time the features, inflections, shared experiences, and unspoken affections that informed our friendships. There was time to tell stories.

In the interim between radiation treatments and starting chemo, I had brunch with our neighbors, the Frishkoffs, and our mutual friends, the Fruchers. We had known each other since 1976. As we enjoyed our meal together, Sandy spoke so beautifully about their trip to the Holy Land that I felt I was there. His words had an immediacy and eloquence that painted the ancient stones gold in the sunlight. They had been awed by the layers upon layers of civilization rooted in the Holy City. As their vivid narrative came to a close, I heard myself saying, "It wouldn't surprise me if one day I, too, walked those sacred stones." Fateful words. Moments later, Sandy spoke privately to me in the kitchen. "Any time you and Andy want to go to Jerusalem, let Floss and me know, and we will cover your fare." A chill went through me and tears came to my eyes at this amazing and unexpected generosity.

Evidently I was still living a miracle. Next year in Jerusalem! The author of my life could not be writing this story to entice me with such a gracious gift only ironically to withdraw it because of resurgent cancer. No. I would live to see Jerusalem. I would pray at the "Wailing Wall"; I would pray, circumambulating the Kaaba; I would pray at the Church of the Holy Sepulchre and along the Via Dolorosa. Gratitude toward life would stream from my lips to God's ears. "Dear Yahweh, Allah the Merciful, dear Lord in whom we live and breathe and have our being—receive our praise and gratitude for the GIFT of life."

When the Lord says, "William, it is time," I go. Until then my heart is set on a pilgrimage to Jerusalem, the New Jerusalem we are called upon to build. The stones of the New Jerusalem are made of Light and Love and Life. Sisters and Brothers, do not be deceived by the pain of passing wars; we are working on building the Temple of Peace.

OUTWARD BOUND

THE THIRTY-THREE DOSES OF radiation therapy extended from December 28 to February 13, with a daily Temodar chaser of 160 milligrams. Then there was a month's reprieve before switching to the 460-milligrams Temodar dose, five days on, twenty-three days off, in a lunar rhythm of twenty-eight days. After conferring with the two doctors closest to us and our situation, Dr. Hertle and Dr. Incao, we determined that I would go by myself (out of the house and across the ocean!) to the Lucas Clinic in Arlesheim for two weeks, followed by an additional two weeks at Casa di Cura Andrea Cristoforo in Ascona. The renowned Lucas Clinic specializes in treating cancer and draws people from all over the European Union. Casa di Cura, on the Swiss-Italian border, treats patients convalescing from a variety of infirmities, including cancer. It had reopened in 2005 after a two-year renovation and expansion. Gift money would cover my airfare and stay. Andy would join me the final week at the Casa di Cura, and then we would have a vacation together in Italy for

three weeks. Was this my swan song, a final farewell to beloved
Italy? Dr. German had responded to our queries about how to
handle the news of the brain tumor: "Take a cruise." We decided
Italy and Italians, with their notorious zest for life, offered the
most nonmedical healing possibilities. Tony and Cory Schifano
clinched the plan by offering us a week with them in Sicily. An
alternative title for this chapter might be "How to Transform
Terminal Cancer into the Vacation of a Lifetime."

Dr. Weaver was skeptical. She didn't want me out of her sight.
I was just about to begin my Temodar treatment at 460 milligrams
per day, the prescribed protocol scheduled to begin a month after
the last radiation treatment. Side effects, complications, intolerance, resurgence, statistics, fatigue, loss of appetite—she has
seen a lot. Couldn't I postpone this trip? But I was intent upon
gathering my life forces to counteract the effects of radiation and
the Temodar chemotherapy. Dr. Weaver is a remarkable person.
She inspires confidence. She is completely frank and direct, pre-
senting clearly the current research, the long odds, and strategies
to deal with recurrence should that become necessary. You felt
better just being in her presence. Was this the best time to leave
the country, she asked? What were these clinics, she wondered?
She was unaware of scientific evidence supporting Iscador treatments. Her main concerns were that nothing should be done that
might interfere with the prescribed chemotherapy. Whatever we
chose to do otherwise was our own responsibility. "You're on
your own." Her warning—to be sure to take the prescribed Glycolax (a laxative) while on Temodar—she impressed deeply upon
me. As if the fear of cancer were not enough, now the fear of
"becoming compacted"! This could be a serious problem, no shit.
I didn't like the sound of it and would take no chances.

I embarked, primed for an adventure in healing. How was I to
know a freak snowstorm would dump two feet of snow in Basel
and I would be stranded in France at Charles de Gaulle Airport?
Exhausted, disoriented, and spaced out, I entered terminal timelessness and found myself incapable of using a phone card.

I had planned to send regular health bulletins to my army of
supporters during my stay at the Lucas Clinic. I was an email

novice with an address book in disarray and superstitious fore-
boding about something called "Mailer Demons." My God! I
just remembered that a worm had snuck into my hard drive and
eaten all my Italian pictures four years prior. I hadn't learned yet
how to back them up or protect against such invasive sabotage.
The precious memories were erased. Significant that this had happened on November 11, St. Martin's Day and Remembrance Day!
Exactly four years later to the day, I had the MRI confirming my
brain tumor, which had wormed its way into the center of my
Mother Board.

A few months later, recovering from surgery and radiation
and far from home, I watched my mass mailing to friends' emails
bounce back one at a time: "error 666," "undeliverable," "address
incorrect," "syntax error." *Syntax*—the word had bad vibes like
a popish plot. Was it possible that random errors and misplaced
periods sabotage my longed-for communication link with my
homeland? How could I uproot the miscreants? What if I was sending multiple copies by trying again and again in a futile attempt
to weed out the bounce-backs? The techno beast was driving me
mad. Would my frustration set off a neurochemical chain reaction
that would reawaken the sleeping monster?

PILGRIM'S PROGRESS

I NEEDN'T HAVE WORRIED. The Lucas Clinic had tech support,
too. Let your shoulders down. "Turn off your mind, relax, and
float downstream." Excuse me, it's time now for my massage.

My missives home, their cyber-wrinkles removed by precision
Swiss technicians told my waiting public all about my adventures
in healing. I've assembled them all into this narrative.

Neither the greatest snowfall since the Ice Age, nor closed
airports, nor downed systems, nor bureaucratic ping-pong, nor

lost luggage, nor phone card babel, nor the hallucinations of sleep deprivation could keep me from my goal: the Lost Clinic of Shangri-la!

Unseen hands opened the door of the Lucas Clinic as I (unencumbered by so much as a tooth brush) approached. SANCTUARY! WARMTH! (Lured by the siren song of nearby Italy and rumors of crocuses in bloom, I had neglected to bring a winter coat). Nurse "Angela" greeted me at the door speaking in melodious English. She showed me to my room: a single with my very own bathroom and feather comforter and pillows. Meanwhile, Mother Holle shook an unending supply of perfectly formed and immaculately clean flakes down (pun intended) from heaven.

Weaving harmonies wafted through lazure-painted halls as my guide led me to the uncommon common room. What was the trio with well-tempered clavier singing as I took my seat among my fellow cancer patients? "Lamb of God, who takest away the sins of the world, have mercy upon us." (If Mr. Carbray had not forced me to learn Latin in high school, I probably would have missed this epiphanic message!) Already feeling blessed enough, by some mysterious arrangement of karma, a friend and fellow patient, Carla Niessen, whom I have known for years, walked through the door. We embraced, happy to see each other still this side of the threshold. There are times you can't tell which side of the veil you're on when you are looking both ways.... Let us revise childhood advice drummed into us for our protection: "Look both ways, before you cross... the threshold."

With music still ringing in my ears, I slept the sleep of the blessed.

MY FIRST LETTER HOME

The joint is clean. Saint Dustin rid the country of dirt and serpents years ago. Spitters have all been deported south of the border. (The squeamish may pass over following paragraph with impunity or opt out of my email list by simply going

to http://www.ispcontrolpanel.com>lukasklinik>shangorill
a>optoutnow.edu. Fill out your consumer-friendly opt-out
registration form. Your Social Security information will be
encrypted automatically to prevent identity theft.) Still with
me? The same Swiss love of order that keeps the trams and
trains on time has devised a scrupulously sanitary, dou-
ble-envelope system for dealing with rectal thermometers
without their coming into contact with fecal (if any) matter.
Or anything else except the location to be monitored. (For
more details, contact the Lucas Clinic directly.) Imagine my
gratitude to my dear informant Terry Morrow, who alerted
me to this system. Try not to imagine my embarrassment
had I not known the routine and naively assumed the same
orifice in common usage on our side of the Great Water
would be involved. Suffice it to say that meticulous notes
are being maintained on more functions than I care to enumerate. *Alles* normal. You gotta love it when, *frisch als der
Morgen der Angela appieren.* (I'm making up this German,
since I don't speak a word. I'm trying to remain inconspicuous in my complete ignorance of foreign languages, but I
have Gringo written all over me. Given the world political
situation, I'm also trying to pass for something benign, like
a Canadian.)...anyway, the nurse comes and says, "How
are your winds?" That's what I call quality care! You can't
get that in the states, because of health care insurance lobbyists and the threat of socialized medicine.

Dr. Lorenz tells Bush jokes. Probably everybody does,
but he does it in English. A great mercy. I'll make it short. St.
Peter is at the gate guarding against illegal aliens (my embel-
lishment). Picasso comes and St. Peter asks him to prove that
he is the famous artist. Picasso draws an incredible picture,
and St. Peter invites him in. Einstein comes. St. Peter asks
him to prove that he is who he says. Einstein writes down his
famous formula, $E=mc^2$; and he is admitted. George Bush
comes. St. Peter says, "I just opened the gates for Picasso
and Einstein. You must prove you are George Bush." "Who
are they?" "Come right in, Mr. Bush."

HOLE-ISTIC & HOLISTIC:
A TALE OF TWO SYSTEMS

THE THIRTY-THREE SESSIONS OF radiation therapy (may affect vanity through hair loss) and Temodar chemotherapy for at least a year is the state-of-the-art allopathic protocaol for my case. Temodar (Breakfast of Champions) is convenient. You can take it at home, but reading the package insert I note that if you inadvertently inhale it, you die. Doctor knows best. The patient then comes in for periodic MRIs until, for one reason or another, they are no longer necessary.

If the tumor should start to get aggressive again (unfair tactics since I've always been a pacifist), they try another chemical in the medical arsenal. The medical establishment offers no Pollyanna projections concerning longevity, morbidity, mortality. Different strokes (pardon the expression) for different folks. Death in the long or short run, however, is guaranteed, with optional afterlives included according to your belief system. Someone said, "We are all dying; some of us just don't know it." I am one of the latter. I may not know who said it, but I get it. Walls of DENIAL erected to defend oneself from fears of abandonment, annihilation, extinction, and the cold void can also dissolve like snow on a sunny day. Cancer will break all barriers. There are two poles of possibility: "I am in a fight for my life against cancer." Or, "Cancer, teach me what I need to learn to change my life. I resolve to work with you."

Still, one must admit that life as we know and love it is terminal (until the next reincarnation, the opt-in program). Isn't it a bit ironic, even uncanny, that we spend more and more time in front of "terminals." Perhaps it is time the anti-radiation shield of the peat vest became standard issue.

From the orthodox medical establishment, one hears a long list of threats and disclaimers concerning what to expect from one's illness. These "facts" are objective, statistical, cautionary, and depressing. A melancholic would assume it's all over, there's nothing to be done. A choleric would fight back. A phlegmatic would placidly take it in stride as long as lunch was on time. A sanguine would book a world tour for several last flings. One of the most sinister side effects in the Chinese menu of dire possibilities I faced, repeated for emphasis, life-threatening in itself, was Temodar's reputed power to stop the *Concorde* in mid-flight. Constipation! Forget prunes! Pull out the big guns: Glycolax (an unwholly owned subsidiary of Mobil or Dow or somebody). Fortunately, I was in Switzerland—Rolex Country—where they understand the importance of regularity.

Communication with the top-of-the-line doctors we encountered at the Albany Medical Center is generally confined to conversations scripted by the legal staff of the hospital and the insurance industry to avoid liability for an ultimately inevitable fact of nature. "Abandon all hope ye who enter" is the undertone. You want hope, you shoulda gone to church, synagogue, temple, ashram, mosque, Stonehenge, or all of the above more often while you still had the time…. Now, it's best to put your affairs in order. Meanwhile, the compassion of the doctors toward the personal situations of their patients remains unspoken but is tangible. They must not create false hope, erring instead on the side of caution. This is a tricky balancing act for a doctor, especially one who recognizes hope as a hugely effective healing force, along with laughter (one reason to be grateful for our President), love, joy, faith, grace, wonder, and the powerful "radiation" of the prayer circle. These life forces and spiritual powers don't fit the grid. They are subjective, anecdotal, individualized, unrepeatable, unpredictable, unscientific, unverifiable, qualitative, and occasionally miraculous. These powers are incommensurate with particle accelerators and transcend actuarial tables. The placebo effect is one of our greatest remedies.

On Wednesday before lift-off to Switzerland, Andy and I went to see my oncologist. I like to say Ankhcologist, since Ankh is the Egyptian word for L'chaim, chi, etheric forces, Life! It was Ash Wednesday. You could tell the holiday after Fat Tuesday, because several of the staff had ashes on their foreheads, signifying a time of fasting, penance, and purification for the forty days preceding Good Friday and Easter. Ramadan and Yom Kippur also have this deeply devotional purpose. Do you ever wish that you could go from one house of worship to another and share in the devotional lives of people of the world who revere the divine sources of life? By synchronicity or cosmic choreography, these same forty days preceding the Resurrection coincided with my time away from Happy Valley. I was expecting Good Friday and Easter to be especially beautiful. My eyes had changed. Mother Earth had already cued the crocuses and snow drops. Buds were swelling in anticipation. Seeds long buried in dark earth will be reborn.

FROM MY LETTERS

I expect to be a New Man when I return, though I may look substantially the same. One can't avoid the daily feeling of living in parallel universes: the bizarre Fast Nacht in Basel with surreally-masked, outlandishly costumed fife-and-drum corps (pardon the expression) parading randomly all over town for four days; moonrise over the snow-capped Goetheanum after Goethe's mysterious fairy tale, "The Green Snake and the Beautiful Lily," told in eurythmy; small talk and table decorum while meeting fellow patients over vegetarian supper, we who have converged at the Lucas Clinic with one key experience in common: our illness/opportunity; and another universe, that of the heart, here and now, in communion with loving thoughts of friends and family back home....

To return to the medical theme (infinite digressions appear to be a side effect of surgery): it was made clear to us at Albany Medical Center that whatever alternative therapies we might choose, we were "on our own." Translation: all the mumbo jumbo and potential quackery (if it looks like a duck and quacks like a duck, we think it's a duck) of complementary therapies were consigned to the at-your-own-risk-not-on-our-watch pile. They are beyond the pale of proven medical science. Not that the orthodoxy has a cure for cancer, mind you, but it will, soon, for urgent humanitarian and commercial reasons. Temodar, by the way, is 500 bucks a pop. Cardiac arrest is another option. Protocols underwritten by alliances of cutting-edge (don't you hate that metaphor?) medical research hospitals and pharmaceutical interests are racing toward the panacea. Pass the stem cells please. Pig hearts for sale. (Hey, I might need one of those, too. I hope he likes French... I mean Freedom Fries.)

The allopathic paradigm understandably focuses on what is wrong. That diseased tissue must be removed. As Occam's razor instructs, "When in doubt, cut it out!" The suspect remainder will be irradiated by the Death Star and death-dealing drugs introduced to interfere with cell reproduction (with apologies to other fun-loving cells and the immune system), because these aggressive cancer cells (insurgents) could crop up anywhere. Rouse the neutrophils and macrophages (think Pac-Man and Homeland Security)! There will of course be some collateral damage in this approach, like the immune system and portions of the psyche (bring on the antidepressants by day and at night the downers). Don't get me wrong; I am grateful for what I have received from this system. But unless you live in an alternative community like Hawthorne Valley, so much healing is locked out. There will come a day when we will have a Lucas Clinic of our own.

To my mind, there is another paradigm that gladly admits the techniques of allopathic medicine while attending to the whole organism both physically and etherically. (More about life forces in a later issue of *Willi's Healing Journey: Catapulted through Illness to La Dolce Vita.*)

Anthroposophically extended medicine not only enlists life forces to restore and retune the individually differentiated etheric body that each of us bears; it also treats the astral, or soul, body, tuning those soul imbalances which have gradually manifested as physical illness because the mobility and fluidity of the etheric body have been compromised. Further, this holistic medical view works spiritually with the relationship of the "I" to health: the mystery of biography, self-knowledge, awakening, inner effort, the capacity of the "I" to penetrate the physical organism. In this holistic context the etheric body, the body of formative forces, is key to sustaining and harmonizing the interweaving systems of the physical body amid the undermining stresses, strains, and environmental hazards (physical and psychological) of contemporary life. Particularly important for many types of illnesses, including cancer, is the interconnection between the "I" and the immune system. *The patient must take active responsibility in the healing process for it to work.*

The philosophical divide between the two systems described poses a root question: Is life built up of molecules ever more complexly arranged (think of lightning striking the primordial ooze) even to the point of self-consciousness; or are life, spirit, and consciousness primary, creating living forms from otherwise-inert matter?

Let medical science wrestle with this dichotomy.

I, on the other hand, heard Bach played on the lute. I KNOW from self-observation that celestial music can retune my instrument. Music therapy is one of several therapies available at the Lucas Clinic.

The Lucas Clinic, where I am now in Arlesheim, Switzerland, specializes in cancer therapy. There are forty-six beds. At the moment there are about thirty patients: Italian, Swiss, German, Dutch, French, and the Lone Gringo. Back to parallel universes. One patient in particular lightens our dinner hour (laughter is the best therapy). Charlotte, who leaves tomorrow after three weeks, glad to be rid of the delicious vegetarian diet, totally uncertain about her future, pulled out a picture from her wallet of herself with Willie Nelson's arm around her. But that's another story. At the Lucas Clinic "Treatment is based on conventional medical knowledge extended by anthroposophy, using holistic methods. It is not a health-cure clinic or a rehabilitation center. Treatment follows clinical necessity." In practical terms, if you are a member of the EU and have health insurance, your medical costs for a stay at the clinic are largely covered! In the USA, devotees of the competitive free enterprise system with dogmatic idealism, standing upon principles of self-reliance, trust the profit motive to stimulate market forces, lobbyists, and big pharma to provide health care or not—devil take the hindmost.

The Lucas Clinic enumerates several reasons for treatment after conventional allopathic techniques have been employed: 1) reinforcing remission achieved with chemotherapy or radiotherapy; 2) treating problems due to tumor diseases; 3) regenerating the damaged immune system; 4) prevention of recurrences; 5) intolerance of conventional treatments; 6) use of special therapeutic measures (i.e., hydrotherapy); 7) treating problems in coping with the disease or adaptation to the implications of the diagnosis.

Who could argue with any of that? But, if the Food and Drug Administration caught wind of the integrative therapies used here, I would be committed to a mental institution, put in the slammer, or be unconditionally cured.

But at the moment I'm too busy to reorganize society into a nation of massage therapists. I don't want to be late for my rhythmical massage. If you should find one day in the Farm Store that someone has placed warm, soothing, fragrant, oleaginous hands upon your shoulders, don't be alarmed. C'est moi, mon cheri! I wish I could convert all but one of my six MRIs ($12,000) into rhythmic massage sessions. The trouble is, there is only one of me (maybe that's a good thing), and the lack of a control group in a double-blind study would demonstrate nothing concerning the respective validity of allopathic vs. complementary medicine in my case. Oh well. In this uncharted territory I am blissfully "on my own." My body, my self—in touch. With a sufficient number of electrodes attached to various brain centers of the subject, me, I believe it could be proven conclusively that rhythmical massage has the power to blow up the equipment!

With a few decisive strokes of the keys, I peremptorily end this email. Expect obscure musings from Casa di Cura Andrea Cristoforo at the foot of Monte Verite overlooking bello Lago Maggiore. If I can't get ultimate answers at a place like that, then fuggedaboudit. I'll just enjoy the view.

Now a word for my sponsors. The prayer circle: Let my gratitude for your loving thoughts toward me stream right back to you.... Now!.... Feel that? That's what I call instant messaging and open access.

Magnifico!

Magnifico! Grazie a Dio! Che bella panorama! Meine Liebe Freunde, In che direzione devo andare? *(Which way do I go?)*

No matter which way I turn, it is beautiful. The Casa di Cura Andrea Cristoforo is perched above the old town of Ascona on the northern shore of Lago Maggiore. To get to the sunny South, the Ticino, from Basel, near the Lucas Clinic, takes about three hours. Smooth, fast, on time Swiss/ Euro-Rail system. The train must climb the Gotthard Pass. (I don't know how Hannibal did it with all those elephants. They don't like going uphill that much, and there was no chocolate at the time to urge them forward.) Since trains have a maximum grade of about fourteen percent, elephants about the same, to gain the elevation, Swiss engineers built a spiral tunnel in the mountains fifteen to seventeen kilometers long about a hundred years ago, chiseled through solid granite. They are a determined folk. Gnomes, however, did most of the grunt work, rolling giant rocks down the mountainside with great glee as they took their schnapps. This was the birth of rock and roll, but it has degenerated into Euro-pop. When the train crosses the great divide, the watershed moment, snow-melt valley streams rush down the slopes (in harmony with ancient Chinese wisdom: "Water flows downhill") toward the great lakes at the foot of the southern slopes of the Alps.

Saturday, a veil of cloud shrouded the landscape, the day of my arrival. Remember late Monet? The painter in his increasing blindness saw in shades of light; no longer objects, but veils of color, nebulous, boundless, mysterious.... I ask myself, "Where am I?" This isn't Kansas anymore. I am suspended between earth and sky.

When I woke the next day, luminous cloud filled the bowl where the lake should be.

The VOID!

From formlessness, gray eminences materialized gradually. Snow-crowned Alps, supposedly solid granite, were now only just perceptible, one with the atmosphere, their solid mass made insubstantial by air. Black birds flying through gray emptiness gave only a vague sense of distance and direction. Who can blame me for being mystified!

Two kind old ladies took me in at breakfast to show me the ropes. Frau Fuchs (or Frau "Fox" as her friend quipped), age ninety-three, and Frau Giovanoli (a mere eighty-eight). I am just a kid, who knows nothing. I used to know a lot, like New York State geography and fractions. But much of what I "knew" has become irrelevant with my sudden change of context. I am more interested in what is behind the twinkle of Frau Fuch's eyes. These ladies are both ageless—youthful spirits with wrinkled fairy godmother faces, filled with the dignity of life experience, wise, gracious, kind, independent, and funny. Frau Fuchs, from Lucerne, reminisced about travels in Algeria seventy years before and about swimming the width of Lake Lucerne, there and back as a young woman. She loved the famous Fast Nacht at Lucerne, when ladies chose their partners. That way you could always pick good dancers! Dancing is different now.... My friends are teaching me Swiss Deutsch and Italian simultaneously. "I will see you tomorrow, God willing," observes Frau Fuchs. No one takes seeing one another the next day for granted.

Our tablemate, Herr Otto (my grandson's name), generously determined to keep conversation alive with a joke, labors in all three languages, including broken English, until I get it. A bear goes through the woods and says to himself proudly, "When I walk, the ground trembles." The lion then comes and says, "When I roar the trees shake and the animals flee." A chicken comes along and coughs. "When I cough, the whole world shakes!"... That's it.... I'm waiting for George Bush to come next, but it's like waiting for Godot. It's over. Oh, wait! I get it! I am like that chicken! I think it's all about me. There is a BIG PICTURE that has nothing to do with my metaphorical cough. I have caught a glimpse of the BIG PIC-TURE as you have held me in your prayers. This is a highly thera-peutic joke. As Frau Fuchs observes, "Laughter is the best medicine." She also shares a proverb "In living, we shall see." Translated from the Latin to Italian, through Swiss Deutsch to me.

Still, despite the kindness of my tablemates, it is not easy for me to be the Lone Gringo. I don't mind listening to conversation, but I prefer to understand what is being said rather than just enjoying the sounds. They do their best to clue me in. I contribute an occasional lame pleasantry, or a noun or two in what I imagine to be Italian or German, like *delicioso* or *Gesundheit,* but it always feels risky and my repertoire is quickly exhausted. I want to say *Offenbarung* or *Erkenntnis,* but they never suit the occasion. I want to crack a joke or say something wise, but don't have the tools. Maybe it is time to blow the dust off of high school Latin and intone *"tempus fugit."* That's profound. As a teenager that phrase always seemed appropriate, but what if I were misunderstood? In any case, a courteous meal under these circumstances can seem . . . . interminable.

I am completely dependent on the kindness of strangers. Frau Fuchs observes that we have developed a "community of table." She suggests we find a name for our club. She is certain that some at other tables wish they were with us. I think she is right.

The food is delicious, as it was at the Lucas Clinic. I had my first fleisch in a long time (not counting the surreptitious donner kebabs in the Basel train station). I have been eating so many vegetables that I may gradually be losing touch with the animal kingdom. My fingers are beginning to look like carrots, my ears like cauliflowers, my head a cabbage. My cheeks are apples. Good for me, no doubt. Muesli and yogurt for morning ballast are washed down with cappuccino (unless you press the wrong button, in which case you get hot milk). The main meal is at lunch with salad bar, soup, vegetarian entrée, and delicious dessert. The evening meal is lighter than midday. Sensible folk. My favorite was a cheese plate with six delicious varieties of cheeses, the omnipresent salad, and panacotta for dessert.

Since it was Sunday when I arrived, there was no doctor's appointment or therapy. After breakfast I descended by a steep and narrow road past the villa-lined cliffs to the town. I was still befogged, but amazed at every turn. Realizing I must return by the same path, the hermetic truth—the way up is the way down—seemed especially relevant. Because the cliffs ascending from the lake are so steep, every tile-roofed villa has its own view of Lago Maggiore (if it is really there), with balconies, terraces, and gardens. Camellias are in full bloom. There are cacti, agaves, palms, pecan trees, cypresses, figs, monkey-puzzle trees, the occasional eucalyptus, ivy-covered walls, ancient wisteria (not yet sprouting), blooming scotch broom, maidenhair ferns, and a host of things I've never seen. The pollarded sycamores at the shores of the lake must be 250 years old. But most significant of all: there is a gingko at the portal of the Casa di Cura. Gingko is known as the Tree of Life. Its relationship to the light forces is such that the veins of its rounded lobe radiate out from the stem or in from the periphery, depending on your point of view. Andy and I, on our first date, the day after we met in the fall of '68, took a sun nap under a Gingko tree in Central Park. Our first date, by "chance" (HA!), was an outing to the anthroposophic bookstore. I had never been there before but felt confident that my pronunciation was correct.... A man mopping the hall said mysteriously, "If you get involved in this, it will change your life." Gingko.

I went to Mass in an old church on Sunday. This was by papal dispensation. No confession required. I, a long-lapsed Protestant, have forgotten what there was to protest about. I'm sure it seemed important at the time. In my present state of grace, I, too, could dip my hand in the holy water and reverently place the sign of the cross upon myself. It doesn't matter that I had been a Jew helping Hiram and crew build the temple; two incarnations prior, a day laborer for the Druids hauling big menhirs and dolmens for religious purposes (unable to foresee that Rolexes would make Stonehenge obsolete). This gave me valuable experience to get hired hauling huge blocks of stone for the pyramids. Someone had to do it. At least by then, we had the inclined plane. But what engages me more is that here at Casa di Cura, it is the reclined plane that allows me to continue my pilgrimage on the astral plane, which does not fit our email format or I would share it with you.

This is the kind of thing that I think about when I dip my fingers in holy water. Now, it was necessary to take off my hat upon entering the *chiesa*. It's cool up there, on and in the dome of my temple with no hat, and, frankly, it looks absurd. I had been sporting a tonsured coif for a number of years, associating it with the opening of my fontanels to receive higher wisdom or a past life regression to my time as a cellular monk. I had not anticipated my hair would simply abandon ship when barraged with radiation, leaving only a shock (I use the term advisedly) of hair, clown-like, front and center. In church either no one seemed to mind, or they began to pray for me, that at the very least my hair might grow back. The jury is still out on how to manage my tresses. My stylist suggests that I take the plunge and choose the Mr. Clean look, accessorizing with a gold earring and possibly a gold tooth. A Harpo or Bob Marley wig would lack the dignity of my former profession and imply a lack of earnestness about my journey. There is a certain purity about the Bruce Willis cue ball. It worked for Brunelleschi, but for the moment, I am sticking with the status quo, waiting for the first signs of spring from follicles subdued by sub-solar radiation.

My therapeutic eurythmist, Frau Ianchi (not Yankee), told me today that a friend with cancer had told her that it is a blessing. "Now a door opens, and I can have a little conversation with God."

My prayers include an expanding circle of friends I have met on this pilgrimage. One prayer envisions a kind of family circle, including spouses, holding hands. That inner circle of mutual support and connectedness, receptive of grace, is surrounded by a much larger circle including you, dear friends, like a Doré engraving of Dante's Paradiso. The innermost circle is shining with the consciousness of "the gift" of our illnesses. Why are we all smiling?

๛

The staff members here are experts. My Dr. Leuenberger is a Mensch. He said something to me so profound about cancer that I refuse to commit it to email.* Only word of mouth for this one. Suffice it to say, it was a cut-to-the-chase moment, and it was a

---

* At this moment, Dr. Leuenberger said, "Cancer is a path to the Christ." It was as if I had been waiting to hear these very words. My heart lifted, and I felt my hope renewed.

good thing. He also said that cancer is our teacher. It has a mission, and those who carry it have a mission. Cancer is teaching us much about our relationship to nature, to the food we eat, to our biographies, to our social relationships, and to our time. It will not go away until we learn what it has to teach.

Gabriella, the art therapist, is wise, witty, insightful, and a pro. She also speaks English, praise the Lord. She went to Emerson College in England thirty years ago. We share a great fondness and respect for Francis Edmunds, founder of Emerson College (small world), who did so much to help Hawthorne Valley get going. I remember only one sentence of the first talk I heard Francis Edmunds give thirty years earlier: "…the education of the will…the will…the will…the WILL." I had never heard anyone repeat a word four times. He hammered it home. After thirty years as a Waldorf teacher and, now, a threshold experience, I know what he was talking about! I will not now begin a pedagogical lecture. I am conserving my forces. But there are deep matters ripening here concerning THE CHILDREN OF THE FUTURE and the education of the will and the heart….

Gabriella has opened the atelier for my use this weekend for clay modeling. That's good. It's raining. The clouds have again settled on the Lago. It is an inward day. Gabriella also led about ten of us in folk songs from the Ticino a couple of nights ago. Songs of love and longing for home. What a scene…our singing together. We went off to bed with an Italian lullaby as our gondola to the spheres.

In addition to *plastizieren,* art therapy, I am continuing my therapeutic eurythmy. At the Lucas Clinic Daniel Marsden was my guide. He and his wife were dear friends of Astrid Barnes. Astrid Barnes was our founding kindergarten teacher. Andy worked for two years as her assistant about twenty-five years ago. Astrid was also a trained eurythmist. After many years of teaching kindergarten, she returned to Dornach to complete her training as a therapeutic eurythmist, a lifelong goal. She practiced her healing art for about two years before her death about ten years ago. I feel her warmth and humor encouraging me to open wide and receive these healing forces. They are a GIFT!

No dissertation, but brace yourself for a few words about therapeutic eurythmy and etheric forces...with apologies to professional eurythmists, doctors, children who wish they didn't have to do it and could play football instead, and all those who have received this email but are encountering the word *eurythmy* for the first time.

The created world is a materialization of cosmic forces. All the forces of light and warmth and life and rhythm and harmony and sound and "chemistry" and "matter" saturate, comprise, form, permeate, regulate, and otherwise come into balance (or not) in visible nature and our own bodies in a continuous process of transformation. We feel these harmonies in our unconscious bodily wisdom, the homeostasis of well being, or we feel out of balance and depleted. But, as the saying goes, there is nothing like a noose around the neck to focus the attention. It turns out that after years of enjoying pedagogical eurythmy, experiencing the benefits for the children and myself, and being led by great teachers gradually, over years, to inner experiences just glimpsing these forces beyond the veil (so to speak), finally I see...WOW! All this is available to me (even me) for HEALING! And everyone can have as much as they like (need) because these life forces are free and everywhere! There are people (trained first in eurythmy, then therapeutic eurythmy, five years total) who can lead me into receiving these energies as they flow through this particular, middle-aged specimen of the human archetype, toward a new balance. The potency is what surprises me.

Rudolf Steiner, referring to Newton's AHA! experience of the apple falling on his head, humorously observed that Newton would have done well to consider how the apple got up the tree in the first place. For that matter, how do billions of tons of leaves unfold with the spring in a breathing alternation of seasons between northern and southern hemispheres? Light, lift, leaf, life, and (dare I say it) love are one fabric. Love it or leaf it. Let's not forget laugh. The predominant focus of our culture on mechanical, gravitational, electrical, and material forces have overshadowed the life forces, the chi, without which we fall to gravity. Here's to levity and the formative forces of the supersensible etheric world, the water of life, the cup of healing!

Some people jog, some do yoga, some swim. I do therapeutic eurythmy. We know the expressions "gather your forces," "focus your energy," "conserve your energy," etcetera. but I now know experientially that the sound-gesture-form of the "U" (as in "blue") streams warmth into my hands and feet immediately. Who turned on the heat? This phenomenon, as one example, is very important for many illnesses, including cancer, because cancer has to do with cold. Steiner, working with the first eurythmists, prescribed a sequence of sounds-gestures-forces-colors-Imaginations specifically for those working with cancer. One of the characteristic features of cancer patients is the tendency to not establish protective boundaries that serve to maintain a balance of one's own energy in relationship to outer demands. (Now they tell me! Could this be you?) The subject generously has a tendency to be too giving (ya gotta remember to look out for number one!) Learning limits is the thing. Now, here comes the power of "B," allowing one to gather forming forces from the periphery, in an embracing, archetypal gesture that is the essence of containment, the boundary between inner and outer, in which the inner space is a column of yellow, enfolded in blue. I'll not go further in futile attempts to describe the indescribable, other than to say that my daily regimen includes a twenty-five minute series of eurythmy exercises for at least seven weeks for it to begin to create lasting benefits. It is so satisfying meditatively that I expect to be doing this work/play for the rest of my now-lengthening life. The prescribed series for me is O, A (as in "say"), M, L, AI (as in "fine"), B, D. Enough! (Holographic, auric color demonstrations are beyond the scope of our primitive, digitized, 2-D technology. Just go to your local therapeutic eurythmist and tell her or him that William sent you. By the way, you need a doctor's prescription. These healing forces are potent and must be wisely directed.)

Andy has come! The sun is shining. The air is claro. Everything is new. Primavera! The camellia festival begins this week.

We will go to the little garden island of Brissago out in the lake and watch the flowers unfold.

Love to you dear friends, Life, and Joy!
Guillermo di Guarda

Return

IT WAS PAINFUL TO leave the Casa di Cura and beautiful Lago Maggiore. In that sublimely beautiful environment well-being streams into the body like the Italian sun. But the journey was not over. Italy itself lay just beyond the frontier. After the rigors of therapeutic message, eurythmy, clay modeling, long naps, afternoon strolls, it was time for a vacation. Who knows if the opportunity would ever arise again? We weren't taking any chances. We would imbibe the artistic (and perhaps culinary) treasures of Italy until we had so saturated ourselves with beauty that our infectious joy and reverence would set Church bells ringing. Why wouldn't we hear bells? After all, we would be there in the Holy Land of Art during Holy week.

With Florence, Venice, and Sicily rounding out the therapeutic journey there was no time for me to email impressions. I just soaked them up, committing them to paper when we returned to the States.

Dear Friends,

Gaunt and weather-beaten, Marco Polo stumbled into Venice in tatters twenty years after his journey to the rising sun and back. He was unrecognizable to family and friends. None believed the wonders he had seen, nor what he claimed to have done. He ripped open the lining of his coat and rubies, pearls, emeralds, diamonds, and sapphires spilled across the table....

We left our protagonist Guillermo reunited with his bride, Andree, on the island paradise of Isole Brissago, floating in the elemental purity of Lago Maggiore. Alps rose steeply above us, the blue ocean of air above them, the generous fire of the sun warming all. The island, formerly the private estate of a Russian Countess, is a Garden of Eden with plants and trees from all over the world.... Emerson (and others) observed: "Plants are the thoughts of God." And that's the way it looked to me.

Primavera was waving her wand. The first Spring of the rest of my life! Withering and dying? No problemo. That's where seeds come in, to bring the new life. How wise. The mother image of each species tucked in a husk that must die to be reborn. "Earth, water, fire, and air/ met together in a garden fair." Natura is now robed in blossoming spring green! Let us not confine ourselves to cars, rooms, and tubes till our senses atrophy. Let us go out into THE GARDEN. At the time of the Flood, the Atlantean catastrophe, Manu had the foresight to bring with him the seeds for the new world. They are still going.

Back to the Casa di Cura. Let us review the array of therapies brought to bear on William's restoration and, dare I say it, resurrection. 1) The Medicine Wheel of sustaining prayers. The healing power of love. 2) Andy's loving, faithful, conscientious, unshakable support. 3) My own ego involvement in my illness and its cure, my positive attitude, my receptivity, my deep conviction that I still have work to do. 4) The help of my guiding angel and wise spiritual beings. My life is in their hands. 5) The insightful guidance of my primary-care physician, Margaretha Hertle, and her knowledge of anthroposophic medicine. 6) Radiation therapy, the death ray, holding at bay the insurgent terrorists lurking in secret cells, guided by Dr. Kim. 7) Chemotherapy to interrupt cellular regeneration periodically so nothing inimical gets a toehold, guided by my oncologist, Dr. Susan Weaver. 8) Iscador mistletoe extract injections boosting the immune system, rallying the troops to guard against illegal aliens. 9) Hydrotherapy, oil dispersion baths of cypress or *lavendula stoechas* (lavender) followed by total relaxation in a cocoon of wool while the absorbed oil releases its potentized etheric forces. Thank you mistress of the baths, Margaret. 10) The healing ministrations of physical therapist Jane Wright. 11) The bioenergetic healing of Zeev Kolman. 12) Music therapy sessions with Gili Lev, concentrating on Bach and Mozart, which ripple deep reverence and abounding joy through my body and soul. 13) Therapeutic eurythmy, now a daily practice. 14) Art therapy, i.e., clay modeling, carving, painting, singing. 15) Dietary support at the Lucas Clinic and the Casa di Cura, a daily life-force smorgasbord of grains, fruits, and biodynamic vegetables. And last, but not least, 16) Rhythmic massage, bless the day I was issued a body. With a full spectrum healing regimen like this, balance has been restored. I am twenty pounds lighter and ten years younger. To Life!

Since rhythmic massage defies verbal description, why talk about it. Just do it. May all your organs, breathing, muscles, joints, meridians, nerves join in the music of the laying on of hands. Receive…receive…receive. "Let the table hold you up." (The opposite of today's refrain "Get a grip.") Paradiso! Whitman had it right, "I sing the body electric!" Rudolf Steiner referred to the sense of touch, out of all the twelve senses (ask if you feel you have been short-changed), as that which is closest to the divine. Hear now the testimony of a man who would not spend a dime to do anything for his body. Tension, carrying "the weight of the world," lockdown, blocked *chi*, stress. Words from the remote past come drifting back. The mysterious Mr. Fremd, my high school English teacher (who died of cancer the year after my graduation) said enigmatically, as I was picking weeds during detention study hall, "Learn to relax." I thought I was! But I have been blind to my body, neglectful of my little donkey who carried me so faithfully and patiently, uncomplaining these many years. Now comes the healing, loving touch of rhythmical massage, the laying on of hands that I too, like the cripple outside the temple, may rise and walk. Only through illness has my carapace dissolved sufficiently to allow this reverent, healing touch to work its wonders. Thank you Nicole, Frau Hagar, and Simon.

On a mythological note, my masseuse at the Casa di Cura bears the surname name Charon, the ferryman who carries us over the threshold between life and death on the waters of oblivion. From these waters of Lethe, one drinks the cup of oblivion, forgetting the trials of earthly existence before entering the Elysian Fields. Rhythmic massage = Elysian Fields. When my body surrenders to therapeutic massage, becoming thought-free, flowing, and receptive, the healing forces common to deep sleep replenish, recharge, and renew the Garden of Eden, the depleted body, to its natural abundant state. The sleep of a baby rocked in the arms of Morpheus. The breath, experienced with inner vision, flows as the winged caduceus along the axis of the spine, penetrating all the organs and enlivening the streaming blood, refreshing every cell as the inner sun crowning the staff fills the body with light. It's a good thing. Thank you, sisterhood/brotherhood of the healing hands.... Thank you, prayer wheel of all paths for sending your help....

The invaluable objectivity of Western medicine informed me that statistically sixty to eighty percent of brain tumor patients with glioblastoma multiforme meet their maker within a year. Temodar extends their prospects on average 2.3 months beyond a year.... But statistics cannot parse the qualitative aspects of an illness which is entirely individualized according to environmental factors, biography, psychological profile, job stress, age, constitution, tumor placement, time of discovery, supportive therapies, etcetera. The first year of survivorship (as I write, I'm at the halfway point) has a negative prognosis. The second year has a "guarded prognosis." By the third year of survivorship the mortality picture opens up for those who made it that far. But the nature of the dormant beast requires vigilance. When my oncologist Susan Weaver said with obvious satisfaction after seeing my latest MRI, "Your condition seems to have resolved itself," there was a moment of jubilation. Bells were ringing. All clear... for the moment. The cancer was quiescent, like the hound of Cerberus. Dr. Weaver was as positive and encouraging as she had previously been cautionary. Meanwhile, the patient continues to bathe in the loving warmth of the extended community and the expert knowledge that has restored my life forces. No wonder I go around hugging people. I'm Jimmy Stewart in "It's a Wonderful Life."

It was not easy to leave the Casa di Cura. The last breakfast with Frau Fuchs ("I see the birds, and I fly inside." "In living... we shall see.") was very poignant. But the journey was not over. Andy's colleagues and many friends had insisted that we have time together as part of the healing journey. This was extremely important for both of us. We were processing a major life change with a BIG QUESTION MARK hanging over our heads. Andy anchored my buoyant feet to the earthly plane, reminding me in the midst of so much beauty that I had not died and already gone to heaven, rewarded by a permanent vacation overlooking Lago Maggiore. No, the story still being written would continue for an unknown period with more revelations, and, no doubt, further challenges.

Still, there was a second honeymoon quality to the remaining three weeks of our journey: Firenze, Venezia, and Sicilia. How could two impecunious Waldorf teachers, thrifty to a fault, parlay serious illness into the trip of a lifetime? The answer is that a circle of generous donors banded together as a private initiative to ensure that we could seek out the complementary therapies that we felt essential, without anxiety about the costs, even if they were not covered by our HVA medical insurance. Are you familiar with an Inuit custom of everyone holding a caribou hide trampoline and flinging high a delighted villager? That's me, in the air.

Through friends' urgings and the great support of Andy's kindergarten colleagues, the therapeutic journey included quality time together as I recuperated from my recuperation at the clinics. We rented a small apartment in Firenze for a week and another in Venezia for a week. Our dear friends Tony and Cory treated us for a week in Sicilia.

It took us a day to reach Firenze, over and through the mountains into the Italian spring. The day began with a cab to Locarno, connecting trains to Belinzona-Milano-Firenze. Cab to apartment. Fifth-floor walkup on a quiet street. Base camp rest. Eight o'clock that evening, we hit the streets to forage for food and found a neighborhood osteria, warm, cozy, authentic with delicious Tuscan home cooking. We slept like logs. We opened the windows the next day and the sun was smiling at us. We had a small balcony where I could do my morning eurythmy exercises overlooking a cubist pattern of red tile roofs largely unchanged from when Dante walked the streets hoping Beatrice would show up. She did! The rest is poetry.

Firenze (Florence), for those a little hazy on their art history classes in college, is the repository for fifty percent of the major artistic treasures of the thirteenth to sixteenth centuries in all of Italia. The explosion of creativity of the Renaissance in all the arts continues to reverberate through Western culture and consciousness. You know the world-weary line from T. S. Eliot: "In the room the women come and go / speaking of Michelangelo...." Any "talk" about Michelangelo, Raphael, Leonardo, Fra Angelico, Botticelli, Donatello is painful before the glory, grandeur, and grace of inspired genius. It is best to be inwardly silent and simply BEHOLD!

Everywhere one turns in Firenze there is a world-famous masterpiece. Emerson said, "Clouds are bread for the eyes," and high art serves the same function. It is nourishment and "music" for the soul. Without imbibing this elixir, life becomes barren, leaving the banal dregs of Gameboy, "reality TV," and shopping. Out on the streets—traffic, commerce, glitz, getting and spending. But in one of the churches, monasteries, or museums of Firenze, it is possible to enter a contemplative sanctuary where the hustle drops away. Here beauty lifted by religious devotion speaks directly, human-divinely, to the creative spirit within each soul.

I feel a didactic episode coming on. We may even cross over into the grandiloquent. Old habits die hard. Bear with me. Beauty is the breath of life. The inspired soul, intoxicated, opens like a flower to the sun, illuminating wide horizons of inner experience. Guided by the intuition, vision, and the unique genius of the artist, inter-weaving powers of colors, forms, harmonies, polarities, rhythms, light and shadow, imaginations and beings lead the entranced observer to sublime realms of wonder, awe, and reverence. Beauty, nature and her "worthiest imita-tor, art," lift the soul from the tomb of habitually con-fined consciousness into day clear light. No wonder, then, that Beauty is the heart of education. In opening the heart, beauty lights the mind and fires the will. This is why all the arts are central to Waldorf education, to all education. The arts, the great educators of humanity, inform the soul life with heavenly human powers through music, poetry, drama, painting, dance, sculpture, architecture, and the "royal art" yet to be realized, the social art. Beauty sculpts the soul. Ugliness hardens it. The deluge of commercialism and technology can submerge love of beauty in a domino effect that also undermines the ability to discern what is Good, and subverts intuition for what is True. In the cur-rent cultural climate of the U.S., questions of education mistakenly revolve around testing, accountability, and tax dollars. This utilitarian myopia to "remain competitive in the global economy" generates great waves of anxiety, stress, and pressure that contort the souls of children like the cruel custom of binding feet. In contrast to this, souls nourished with beauty become fountains of creativity whose abundance waters culture like spring rain on bar-ren fields. Children, break your #2 pencils, do not fill in the bubbles. Instead, drink from the wellsprings of imagination, jump into the fountain of beauty!

Enough tirade. We resume our journey. Andy and "eye" cruised the galleries, naves, cells, palazzi, crypts, domes, cathedrals, chapels, and cloisters examining mosaics; reliquaries; vestments; frescoes; tapestries; sculptures of bronze, wood, and marble; carvings of ivory; sacramental vessels; fountains and gardens until we were saturated or brain-dead, whichever came first. Then we would have a delicious late Tuscan lunch followed by a well-deserved nap with visions of Raphaelic cherubs on cloud nine while the myriad impressions sorted themselves out. What would we do without the unconscious to sift through our virtual slide collection? Then we would jolt down an espresso and hit the streets. If I attempted to tell you what we saw, I would never finish this summation of our journey. We did all that was humanly possible without undermining my steadily reviving health. Beauty therapy was the strategy, and it works.

The streets. Endlessly fascinating. No one is at home watching TV (what's that?), or reading a book (lonely occupation). Everyone is talking. The music of the Italian language is an effervescent fountain: rhythmical, dramatic, joyful, passionate, operatic, effusive, contentious, rhetorical, outgoing, cordial, expressive, explosive, and dulcet by turns. Who knows or cares what they are saying? Maybe they don't even know. Everyone is talking at once. Everyone has a cell phone. Hands are dancing, gesticulating, shrugging, bargaining, waving, signifying, coaxing, caressing, greeting, offering, suggesting. The *passagiato* (evening promenade) is in full swing. People on parade. Pedestrians only. All ages: peacocks, wolves, chicks, goats, roosters, fillies, monkeys, fashionista babes, cruising raggazi, bambini, dignified signori, touristi, African street vendors, indulgent Grandmas, silk merchants, street musicians, nuns, beggars. Glittering, glitzy windows sparkle with costume jewelry, garish colors, provocative designer fashions, the pointiest of cowgirl boots, the Armaniest of Italian suits, kinky mannequins, astronomical prices.

Two archetypal/religious themes emerged with the greatest relevance and immediacy for us in the context of my illness and path of healing: the Mother of Mercy, Mary, and the death and resurrection of Christ. The rebirth of nature, Passover, Palm Sunday, Good Friday, and Easter Sunday coincided with our time in Italy. Who am I not to get religion? Everything spoke of the sacred joy of life, the mystery of death, and the hope of healing. There we were, surrounded by holy images, miracles and mysteries that resonated so profoundly with our personal journey through the Valley of the Shadow of Death. "There are no atheists in the foxholes." Meditative prayer in each of the sanctuaries we visited deepened into true communion with the spiritual sources that alone could heal me. I always felt supported by my friends' loving thoughts toward my recovery, as I also sent my prayers toward my new friends from the clinics who were also working with cancer.

For the past several years Andy has been making a special study of Mary, Mary Magdalene, Sophia, Demeter-Persephone, and Isis. The Holy Mother and Child image looked compassionately on us from every church we entered. Always, the most votive candles were burning in her chapels. It is the realm of the Great Mother, the Mother of mothers, the Eternal Feminine, the divine Sophia-Mary that is entrusted with the birth and nurture of the Holy Child. Her receptive, innocent soul accepts the spiritual mandate to become the earthly vessel that gives birth to the Son of Man. It is not possible in this therapeutic travelogue bulletin to do more than allude to experiences of gratitude, grace, and mercy that occur in the inner sanctum of the soul. Nor is it right to be completely silent about it. We need not attempt to compare the relative effectiveness of radiation therapy and Andy's lighting of candles for me in front of miraculous icons of Mary and the Holy Child. Both approaches have their effective virtues. Love lights life.

Even fleeting thoughts that occur in the midst of shopping and driving, "I wonder how William's doing?" are woven into the fabric of warmth that wraps around me.

Before leaving Firenze we found again the centuries-old apothecary attached to the cloister of Santa Maria Novela. Four years before we had stumbled on this historic dispensary of the Dominicans' knowledge of medicinal plants. This knowledge of healing flows in continuous lineage dating back as far as Hermes Trismegistus and includes such contributing luminaries as Aesclepius, Hippocrates, Gallen, the Druids, the Cathars, the Therapeutae, Averroes, Avicenna, Paracelsus, the herb gatherers and persecuted midwives of the Middle Ages, anonymous alchemists, and the miracle healers of the Christian tradition. The rococo ceilings of the apothecary are variously frescoed with a great healer from each continent in a brotherhood/sisterhood of herbal and chemical knowledge that includes a New World shaman, a Sybil, Mercurius, an African tribal doctor, et al. Old mortars and pestles are on display along with retorts, alembics, "pelicans," and distilleries. Wonderful aromatic salves, ointments, compresses, compounds, digestives, and elixirs are there for any ailment, along with soaps, cosmetics, and essential oils.

This was not CVS or Eckerd's, densely populated by a bewildering array of synthetic drugs with litanies of side effects. No, this was in the stream of healing that perceives the relationship of the stars, the sun, the moon and the planets to the organs, rhythms, and functions of the body and understands that the macrocosm reveals the spectrum of substances from meteoric iron to mistletoe to formic acid needed to sustain the balance of life in human form.

Arrivederci Firenze, buon giorno, Venezia! Venezia is a dreamscape. It is so magnificent, improbable, ornate, exotic, grand, opulent, "other," that it is incomparable. There are no cars in the city itself. This is huge! Not to be swamped with sound. It is a quiet city. How can you tell what century you are in? The downside is that it is so uniquely beautiful that twelve million visitors come annually for a look (most of them for a day or two...good luck.)

If you avoid the prime tourist route between the Rialto Bridge and St Mark's Square, you can easily lose the crowds and get lost in the quiet, charming neighborhoods and small canals of this labyrinthine city. In fact some people get so lost they never come out. We stayed in an off-the-beaten-track neighborhood in the Castello quarter near San Pietro di Castello with its leaning tower. Here we celebrated Mass, Palm Sunday morning.

A wooden bridge over one of Venezia's innumerable canals connected us with the conglomeration of lagoon islands that comprise the canal city of Venice. It was a twenty-minute walk from our little ground floor apartment to the Doge's Palace and Piazza San Marco. One is walking through a living architectural, cultural museum spanning a millennium from the days of Byzantium (Constantinople-Istanbul) through the Napoleonic invasion. Venezia Serenissima! The independent Republic of Venezia held the delicate balance point between the Eastern Orthodox Church of Constantinople and the Catholic Church of Rome. It was an unrivaled naval and mercantile power of incredible wealth, controlling and protecting East-West trade. The navy was its homeland security. In the heyday of its strength as a sea power, unbelievably, it could crank out a naval vessel a day in its shipyard, the Arsenale, manned by three hundred marines at the oars, citizens, not slaves, ready to engage the Genovese or Turkish enemy or transport the Crusaders to the Holy land.

The city is built on pilings driven into the shallow waters and mudflats of the lagoon. The ninth-century Basilica San Marco alone is supported by a million such piles. Its marble mosaic floors are rippled with the effects of time and water in supporting such an exquisite edifice. As you know, Venice is endangered by high tides and climate change. Periodic flood tides turn Piazza San Marco into a reflecting pool. The city is "subsiding." The world refuses to let it sink.

According to legend, San Marco, in his travels spreading the Gospel, had a vision that his final resting place would be where Venezia is now. Nine centuries later, when Venezia was considerably more than mudflats in a shallow lagoon, Venetian merchants fulfilled the prophecy by absconding with the body of St. Mark wrapped in a rug. The Basilica San Marco was built in his honor. This is one of the most magnificent buildings in the world. The multicolored marble columns, the beautiful domes, the statuary, and the exquisite architectural tracery of the exterior in the Byzantine style are magnificent. But inside... gold mosaics cover every inch of the domes, telling stories from Creation to Resurrection. Totally astounding! So is the magnificent inlay of the marble floor. From 1075 on, every ship returning from abroad was required to bring back a gift to adorn the house of San Marco. This building was designed to waft one up to the seventh heaven.

When the visitor emerges into the light of day amid throngs of people distributed over the football field-sized piazza, the dreamscape of the city is still there. Look where you like, the Palazzo Ducale (Doge's Palace), the Grand Canal, the beautiful churches and bell towers, the gondolas, the arcades, merchants' palazzi vying in grandeur—it's a phantasmagoria. Time to sit and absorb the spectacle before it vanishes into the coral atmosphere of the Venetian sunset, dreams, and fond memory.

Instead of buses, the Venetians and tourists use the vaporetti, the narrow, shallow draft boats that continuously ply the canals. The cruise from one end of the Grand Canal to the other, past all the palazzi and under the Rialto Bridge, takes about forty minutes, zigzagging across the canal to various stops. Circumnavigating the cluster of connected islands takes an hour. After such a ride, the rocking of the boat stays in the legs for hours, on into sleep. The canals get into your blood.

The Pescheria and the Erberia adjacent to the Rialto Bridge are a trip. Calamari, pulpi, red snapper, sea bass, tuna, mussels, anchovies, *gamberini* (shrimp), you name it, they've got it. I don't think you can buy a frozen fish in Italy. This is the day's catch on ice. Gift from the sea. The Rialto vegetable markets right next door are a rainbow of fresh produce. There is haggling for the best price, part of the fun, but to the Italian consumer food is religion. Mama knows. Shopping is not loading a cart with processed convenience foods. The market is a ritual, the sacrament of *abbondanza*, a celebration of Natura's cornucopia. Genetically modified food? Don't mess with Mother Nature. Also wonderful are the flower and vegetable boats that bring the produce to the neighborhoods.

I will not bore you with a travelogue of sights you can find in any guidebook. But I must mention Scuola Grande di San Rocco. Tintoretto painted the interior. The Scuola was a charitable brotherhood dedicated to San Rocco who devoted his life to healing the sick. The brotherhood wanted something special. An artists' competition was held for preliminary drawings for the first commission. While other noted artists submitted wonderful ideas, Tintoretto, in a hurricane of creativity, proposed a design for the entire hall (think Grand Central Station or the Sistine Chapel). He struck a deal. He would do the whole thing. All he wanted was a commitment of a hundred ducats a year and no further judgments among competing artists, so he could realize this comprehensive vision. This was to be a labor of love extending for two decades out of the depth of his devotional life. He would do about three of these huge paintings per year. Stylistically, he started where Michelangelo left off. In the course of time he completed about fifty of these paintings. Henry James said of the *Crucifixion*, "No single picture contains more of human life; there is everything in it, including the most exquisite beauty."

Moses Strikes Water from the Rock, The Miracle of the Bronze Serpent, and *The Fall of Manna in the Desert* celebrate the intentions of the Scuola in alleviating thirst, sickness, and hunger. These tempestuous paintings contain hundreds and hundreds of people depicted with every conceivable variant of emotion and dramatic gesture at crisis moments of divine intervention into biblical history. This was the polar opposite of the serenely beautiful, contemplative frescoes of Fra Angelico in Firenze. Tintoretto was a man on fire. Even his brushstroke was fevered and impressionistic. It amazes me how dismissive I had been to this mannerist style before now. The same goes for Titian whose inspired vision of the *Assumption of the Virgin* is right next door. I once was blind, but now I see. Beauty, like gelato, comes in many flavors.

I will not mention the Peggy Guggenheim collection, the Accademia, the Palazzo Ducale, the glass-blowing artistry on the island of Murano, the twelfth-century Romanesque church (also on Murano), the innumerable lion sculptures throughout the city, the naval museum, the omnipresence of elaborately artistic Carnival masks available for sale, or anything else, because it's over and I have to get on with my new life.... But Sante Maria della Salute cannot be overlooked. This church was built to give thanks to Mary for the miracle of saving the city from a plague that decimated Venezia in 1630. To this day, in November, a candlelight procession across a bridge of boats to the sanctuary honors her intercession. The harmoniously proportioned church is of white marble, a pillared octagon with tall portals and graceful dome at the entrance to the Grand Canal. A statue of Mary crowns the capital. Sunset turns the church into a lovely rose reflected in the dancing waters of the canal. *Salute* means health and salvation. Thank you Mary, Mother of Mercy, for watching over Venezia and us.

On to Sicilia! We arrived at 8:00 p.m. Stepping off the plane, we were immediately intoxicated with the scent of orange blossoms that succeeded in drowning out the jet fuel. We knew we were on the right track. Our dear friends Tony and Cory picked us up in every respect. Tony is of Sicilian ancestry. His delight at being for the first time on his native soil was radiant. To celebrate this "homecoming," Tony, a car connoisseur, rented an Alfa Romeo for our collective comfort. Think autostrada speed, hairpin turns on narrow mountain roads with oncoming buses, Gran Prix maneuverability into the Centro of old cities, flying entirely by some ancestral wisdom and a black belt's reflexes. The unflappable Cory, with infallible sense of direction and split-second intuition, navigated while Andy and I enjoyed the scenery. We arrived at our suite (they had given us the front room, must have been part of the therapeutic plan), with expansive shared terrace in the east coast beach town of Leto Janni. We ate a celebratory dinner at 10:00 p.m., not embarrassingly early like most English-speaking tourists. Then we crashed.

Easter morning, the Resurrection! And where were we? On the ancient island of Sicily, in the Mediterranean Sea, within striking distance of the active volcano Mount Etna, surrounded by rocky cliffs, amidst blooming shrubs and wildflowers of all hues. We went to Easter morning Mass together. Tony had been an altar boy. He knew Catholicism from one side and has some issues with the Church. I had grown up as Episcopalian (until old enough to resist) and shined my shoes and said my prayers (heaven help me if I should forget anybody), and I was very concerned to hear about Purgatory, Limbo, and Hell from my Catholic neighbor. Cory had been brought up in a younger, free-thinking generation and had little experience with formal religion, much less indoctrination. And Andy had grown up in the Bible Belt, gone to a Presbyterian Church when young, but didn't have no truck with anything like the papacy, Evangelical Christians, New Agers, gurus, and such like.

In the eye of the storm of my illness, an understanding for the importance of Mary and Mary Magdalene and Sophia has become increasingly meaningful and necessary both on a personal and a macrocosmic level. The straight-jacketed soul longs for the transformation of consciousness from patriarchal, militaristic, imperialistic, egoistic dominance toward a culture closer to nature, filled with compassion, love, interdependent support, healing, and peace. The heart knowledge of the Mother of Mercy, which all women possess as intuitive wisdom, will be balm for the unbridled competition so prevalent in a male-dominated world. The male soul also longs for this release, peace, and gentleness. On this Easter morning, gratitude for my illness and our journey; a profound feeling of grace, thankfulness and prayers for fellow patients on the way; warm acceptance of all the help I have been receiving; deep love of family and friends; and hope for the future blended in joyful renewal. Peace be with you. He is risen!

Outside the packed church, the morning light was especially brilliant. The sea air itself was celebratory. We walked on the beach and stuck our toes in the baptismal water of the Mediterranean. The polished wet pebbles shone with individual character, each with ancient stories to tell. Even my freshly shaved head gleamed like Brunelleschi's Dome or a giant Easter egg. Everything fit together. All will be well.

It is time to conclude these notes. For the sake of brevity, I will not say anything about the looming majesty of Mount Etna, the picturesque streets and amphitheater of Taormina, the ancient Valley of the Temples of Agrigentum, the glory of the Sicilian landscape in spring, ruined Norman forts, the vertiginous mountain towns, the coves and cliffs of Isola Bella, dining late by the sea on delicious Sicilian cuisine, the taste of zuppa de pesche with a glass of Prosecco, watching the constellations pass the time, and the joy of friendship which I share with all of you.

At his grandfather's urging, little Tony would climb the precious fig tree in Queens. The figs were at the peak of ripeness, like fruit from the Tree of Life. From ground level grandfather would call up, "Not for the bowl. *Eat the fig!*"

How sweet it is, so full of life.

> Love, Light, Life
> Your friend,
> William

VITA NOVA

WHEN I RETURNED FROM my Therapeutic Journey, I was a New Man—in process. In the six months since surgery, tools had been given me to work with: the oil dispersion baths, Iscador treatment, and therapeutic eurythmy were powerful stimuli toward full recovery. Though my life forces had taken a hit, my resolve was to build them up in a new way.

Cancer had cracked the nut of habit. The sprouting seed of my recovery, long buried in earth, was growing again into life and light. My "irrational exuberance" at resurging vitality was irrepressible. Fortunately, I regained the ballast of life's sensible rhythms: things like morning coffee and granola, writing, making lunch, the necessary midday naps, shopping at the Farm Store, afternoon walks, assisting Andy in preparing the evening meals, talking with visitors. My "work" was rest, relaxation, and rejuvenation. The dominant mood underlying my buoyant normalcy was "I am alive!" This was a fragile respite, easily overturned, therefore all the more precious.

"You look younger," commented surprised friends. I was younger. The metamorphosis was still in process, radiating from the inside out. I was more present, more attentive to little things: light in the trees, contours of the land, shades of lichen, crunch of leaves, the green health of moss, changing hues in sunsets, the tone of people's voices, their expressions and soulful eyes, the vivid color and taste of food, the flight of birds.

Solitude was crucial. My mind was not whirring and wanting as it had been. The pond was still. I could drink in the "suchness" of now. I was liberated from acquiring, adding, gaining, figuring out. I had crossed over into the land of what is, IS. I confess that I had the subtle feeling of not being alone. As wistful thoughts drifted through my uncluttered mind, my wondering gaze found companionship in the smallest delights. Delicate perceptions long ignored came forward out of the trees to see who I might be when left to myself. Was Natura enjoying my enjoyment of her beauty? I should ask and listen.

"Exceptional dew you have today, dear Lady," I thought to myself. "It sparkles in the grass like little suns."

I've been waiting for you to wake. I knew you would love the scattered dew jewels. Do you see how legions of my spider fishermen have cast their nets for the new day? They are catching nothing but pearls.

"How patient and alert they are ... dear Lady, everywhere I look I see newness. Have you always been so radiant?"

Did you forget, my child?

"Help me remember now, dear Lady."

Could it possibly be that appreciation for the particular gesture of a tree, close examination of unfolding buds, delight in the chirps of spring peepers, the soothing sound of April rain, the birth of robins outside my window were all mysteriously carried as a loving light-stream of consciousness back to the Matrix from which all flowed? I drank from the spring of delicate delight in Natura, and she quenched my thirst with daily reawakening to her beauty and fullness. Morning forays into the nuances and mysteries of Mother Earth modestly and minutely disclosed nature's script in the Garden of Life. Was my gentle enthusiasm and warm interest fulfilling the veiled world's longing to be known and loved? Are we human beings the doors of perception through which creation wakes to the spectrum of its glory? Or must we be cut off from our subtler experiences, clueless, careless, the last to see?

A cacophony of interior protest scatters and ridicules all deeper connection with the beings of the natural world: no Gnomes allowed. Living nature? Give it up. Impossible. Quaint. Lunacy. Throwback. Pathetic Anthropomorphizing. Laughable. Unscientific. Superstitious. Delusional. Subjective. Creepy.

Still, the longing to penetrate into the core of nature persists. No longer estranged, may I receive the loving embrace of Primavera, the bride? "Hear me shy forest friends, you elemental spirits of earth, water, air, and fire. I need your wisdom to find you again, to know how to be with you. I have forgotten all I once

remembered when the world was new. Teach me again to be playful, receptive, participating, recognizing, appreciating, attending,
and opening. Teach me, animate nature, how to enter in."

Who calls to me in all this abundant being? The shy, hidden
ones of gnomish stone, wavering leaves, airy breath, shimmer of
water, glimmer of light whisper expectantly.

*Shhhh. Friends, here he comes on his walk. Places everybody.
Let's see what he sees today. Just try to act natural, be relaxed, at
home in the world. Don't get your hopes up too high, but today
might be the day we will be discovered....*"

Always I am rewarded with a small gift from a walk in the
woods: the smallest treasures of mosses in miniature perfection,
of sprouting buds and moldering humus, of an inconspicuous
unnamed blossom, or scurrier on beetly business. Being fills
every crevice.

HALLELUJAH SIDE

*When we get home there will be no dying,
when we get home to glory land,
I am living on the Hallelujah side.*

INCORPORATING WHAT I HAD been learning was a continuing
process. By "incorporating" I mean literally remaking the substance of the physical body. I was open for repairs, undertaking
extensive remodeling. Cancer patients have ups and downs, good
days and bad days. This is complicated by the existential ele-
ment of suspense for the patient and loved ones that dictates a
ride on an emotional roller coaster, just when equilibrium is most
essential. But I was in an expansive grace period. I felt strongly
that there was purpose behind my good fortune — meeting cancer, learning much, surviving so far. This providential day-to-day

living, bucking long odds, was worth celebrating. I longed with all my heart, in comradeship with my growing circle of cancer friends, that this ark would raise us all up by the grace we were all receiving. Since I had evidently been given a cup of healing, I wanted to share it with everybody. I was not blind to the suffering and fear that comes with a diagnosis of cancer. Far from it. But I was driven by the urge to find a way to convey facets of my experience and a sense of direction that would be solace, service, and hope for others in dire need.

Even my own fortuitous reprieve from death could be withdrawn without prior notice. Who knows? As Frau Fuchs, my wise table companion at the Casa di Cura, says, "In living we shall see." I could offer friendship to fellow travelers, but what counsel was I qualified to give to anyone else? What was unique to my situation? What might be more broadly shared among others in the same boat?

One thing I knew, the survivor's relationship to life and death is irrevocably changed. The same is true for the survivor's family. Walk a mile in my shoes to know what I mean. Cancer has two primary aspects. One is the Gorgon, the dreaded foe, the writhing beast, the devouring maw. The other aspect of our illness bears the elixir of healing, the intention of which is spiritual healing, transformation, courage, mercy, reconciliation, peace. With its help, we are to forge, proactively, a new relationship to life *and* to death. Then we will discover the deeper wellsprings of both. Can the individual struggling with this illness find the spiritual courage to embrace with equanimity the reality of death? Can we hold death in the light? This depends on plumbing the depths of soul. Is death for you extinction, darkness, the void, torment, fear of oblivion? Or is approaching the end of one's life an opening, letting go, release, and the birth into the spiritual world? Your rabbi, priest, minister, doctor, spiritual counselor, hospice worker, or friend may help you with wise words and prayers. But, ultimately, each of us "will walk that lonesome valley by ourselves."

In our search for life forces, let us take a leaf of grass from Walt Whitman:

> Come, lovely and soothing Death,
> Undulate round the world, serenely arriving, arriving,
> In the day, in the night, to all, to each,
> Sooner or later, delicate Death.
>
> Prais'd be the fathomless universe
> For life and joy, and for objects and knowledge curious:
> And for love, sweet love—But praise! praise! praise!
>
> For the sure-enwinding arms of cool-enfolding Death.
> Dark Mother, always gliding near, with soft feet,
> Have none chanted for thee a chant of fullest welcome?
> Then I chant it for thee—I glorify thee above all;
> I bring thee a song that when thou must indeed come,
> come unfalteringly.
>
> Approach, strong Deliveress!
> When it is so—when thou hast taken them, I joyously
> sing the dead,
> Lost in the loving, floating ocean of thee,
> Laved in the flood of thy bliss, O Death…

Life steers us now in an unfamiliar direction. Despite fear, we learn to embrace Death with courage, as we embraced life with joy. We release the remnants of avoidance, denial, anger, or fear. Step by step we make the ascent through acceptance, patience, deep listening, and forgiveness. In death, illness is transmuted to release, sorrow to blessing, loss to gratitude, death to awakening.

The word *patient* characterizes only the passive side of receiving help. The active side of the inner journey continues through all obstacles as this verse by Rudolf Steiner conveys:

> To us it is given
> At no stage ever to rest.
> They live and they strive the active
> Human beings from life unto life
> As plants grow from springtime
> To springtime—ever aloft,
> Through error upward to truth,
> Through fetters upward to freedom,

Through illness and death
Upward to beauty, to health and to life.

The gift of life that I have received, that we all receive, comes
from opening heart, mind, and hand, not clutching. As a gift, life
is not "mine" anymore than my oxygenated blood is "mine" or
the air I inhale and exhale is "mine." We move in the being of
the superabundant cosmic generosity of Life flowing through us
as bountifully as sunlight. This is the Life in which we live and
breathe and have our being. Let's take another taste, now, while
it's on our mind. Ahhh. L'Chaim!

We will return this gift of life, inhaled at birth, as we exhale
soul and spirit at death. The physical body returns to earth,
Whitman's compost heap, from which the leaves of grass spring
eternally. And the etheric forces return to the cosmic ocean from
which they came. Soul and spirit continue their journey through
soul and spirit lands. Don't take it from me. What do I know?
Just wait and see and prepare to be surprised. But for here and
now, trust me, nourishing reverence for death is as important as
cultivating reverence for life. They are sister and brother.

From my small corner of the planet with its 3.5 billion souls
coming and going, my personal mandate has become clear. The
more light and love I give and gratefully receive, the more becomes
available for others to share. I am a *soular* collector. I am a generous generator. I am a *soular* cell in the body social. When I am
unable to contribute what I can on this side of the threshold, I will
do what I can from the other side. That gift will be more than we
know at present. There will also be laughter coming from that
quarter over our myriad illusions on this side. And there will be the
deepest earnestness as we grow resolute for our ongoing voyage.

It gives me joy to think,
I'm gonna to take a trip
In the ole' Gospel Ship
I'm going way beyond the sky
I'm gonna shout and sing
Until the heavens ring
When I bid this old world good-bye.

Now that I think about it, I have a fitting repertoire of songs for the occasion of my passing when it comes. Truth to tell, I've been preparing for this day all my life. "Glory, glory, hallelu-jah! / Since I laid my burden down." You know the tune, it sings itself, just join in and improvise to your heart's content. I expect to be singing in the heavenly choir nightly with you, brothers and sisters. That's where we get the joy juice for the next day.

> When we've been there ten thousand years
> Bright shining as the sun
> We've no less days to sing God's praise
> Than when we've first begun.

Children of the Future

Flashback to Scrooge the tightfisted, cold-hearted, shadow of a human being. Only when he kneels beside his own grave is he moved to heartfelt repentance. He vows to become a new man: "I will honor Christmas in my heart and try to keep it all the year. I will live in the Past, the Present, and the Future. The spirits of all three shall strive within me. I will not shut out the lessons that they teach."

Like Scrooge, our withered worldview has become too egocen-tric and ossified to overcome the weight of its own self-importance. As individuals and as a culture there is a longing for a change of heart, of outlook, of intention, of consciousness.

The temptation to enumerate the things that need transfor-mation in our society is so strong that there is a kind of fiendish pleasure in indulging it. Beware. That would only add to the gravity weighing us down. Breathe. Believe. Be. Playful, prayer-ful levity leavens and enlivens the fallen and leaden, lifting our lives like leaves into light and life in the sun of love resplendent in heaven.

Children of the Future, Welcome! You sow the new seeds of Heart and Will that sun-ripen into Living Thinking. Dead thinking, the counterfeit image of our narrow conception of ourselves, falls away as an empty husk. The generation of children now streaming toward earth is filled with Life, Love, and Light in such abundance that we rediscover our own, emerging humanity waking from enchanted sleep.

The pendulum of materialism and spiritual blindness has swung to the breaking point of brittle, outmoded thought forms. The frozen ice is breaking up. Seed forces of renewal are cracking the concrete and springing to irrepressible life. Joyful and compassionate and strong-willed children, guided by wisdom and love, hold the spiritual intention to work for the transformation of the world. Now.

Who am I to make such blanket, unsubstantiated assertions? I am, like you, Mother-Father, gazing into the open face of your joyful newborn child. In the eyes of the child, we realize we have always known one another. Our mutual recognition and mirroring love is a freely given offering and a vow. We offer you reverence, devotion, protection, and encouragement to help each and every new "I" fulfill the path of her and his becoming.

"And a child shall lead them." We will rediscover ourselves, our Selves, to the degree that we recognize these Children of the Future and their gifts. This awakening has to do with the Holy Child, the Inner Child, Every Child. The Child bears a perpetual gift for humankind. LOVE is the GIFT. The more it is given away, the greater it grows. Gradually awakening humanity is still at the beginning of a long evolutionary process of receiving and sharing this most generous GIFT, from our highest Self to all Children of the Future.

We have a long climb ahead. We are slaves still, fettered to our prejudices, our desires, our will to dominate, our egotism, our materialism, our blindness, our fears, our projections, our demons, our history, our greed, our crippling self-image, our sorrows. So encumbered, how can we recognize our radiant selfhood? The Holy Child will touch our eyes with healing love. The joy of our release will lift our voices in song: "I once was lost, but now I'm found, was blind, but now I see." See what? The whole, Holy Human Being, in the full light of day.

But we have to prepare ourselves to receive the blessing of discovering the Holy Child in our midst. Overcoming the weight of centuries, we must lift our gaze to the hills, the mountaintop, to the sun, to the stars finally to remember where we come from and who we truly are. This deed of self-discovery opens the doors for the Children of the Future to offer their abundant gifts into the world.

Do you like stories? All children do. The Child of Good Fortune, who is each one of us, is cast upon the Waters of Life, like Moses, like Osiris. Each of us undergoes trials to earn the wisdom—the gold of life and love and light—before we can marry the princess. O Happy Day! However, the princess wants nothing to do with marrying a scruffy commoner. We must win her heart through deeds.

To gain her love, the Child of Good Fortune must go the other direction and descend to the Underworld to pluck three golden hairs from the Devil's head. This is facing death with courage. Fortunately, the Wise Old Lady, the Devil's grandmother is there to help. The task of plucking these golden hairs from the Devil's head teaches the Child of Good Fortune all he needs to know to renew the world.

The Child learns he must free the ferryman who took him to the shore of the nether world. This sad soul is bound to go to and fro eternally until he can let go of his sticky oar. The Child must kill the mouse that chews the roots of the tree that used to bear golden apples. Then the Child must kill the frog that chokes the spring that used to flow with wine. When the fountain flows with wine again, and the Tree of Life again bears golden fruit, and the ferryman is free, then the Child of Good Fortune unites in marriage with his bride. This is the long-awaited union of Soul and Spirit, wholeness, Holiness, Selfhood. The evil king, who did everything within his power to make the Child fail or die, justly becomes bound to the sticky oar, his own greed and egotism.

Every Child who hears this ancient story (collected by the Brothers Grimm) listens with the deepest attention, with the profoundest identification. They know this is a map, a blueprint, and a key to the treasure of the Self. They will find their way over, around, under and through all the challenges of life to their higher Self, their true humanity.

The Children of the Future, like the Child of Good Fortune, in their openness to life have enhanced capacities to enter whole-heartedly into earthly existence, each in her/his own individual way. With grace, guidance, and good will they will fulfill the tasks of their unique spiritual intentions. Like the harmonic structure of the Medicine Wheel surrounding the Holy Child, Every Child has her or his own place in the circle of united will to give birth to resurging humanity. Angelic help will be given them to share the mosaic of their gifts. Strengthening challenges will also abound.

Are we open to receiving the gifts brought by the Children of the Future? Can we nurture the wholeness that makes them Holy? Failure to recognize their gifts condemns them to never realizing their royal destiny. They must not fall prey to the monotonous passage of time going to and fro, never to taste the golden fruit, never to drink the wine that freely flows from an inexhaustible fountain, never to win through to awakened Selfhood.

Without realizing it, we all bear aspects of the evil king that would thwart the Child at every turn. In speaking for myself, perhaps I speak for others. I have held that oar of back and forth monotony, repetitive and dutiful effort without delight. I recognize in my own busyness and nervousness that nibbling mouse forever gnawing on the roots of the Tree of Life. I have experienced the thirst since the fountain that once flowed with wine has dried up.

But then the Child of Good Fortune freed me! We, too, will be set free by the Children of the Future. But we must earn our freedom.

All we have to do is pluck three hairs from the Devil's head. It's child's play. Choose a Devil ripe for the plucking. I have my own candidates. However, if the Devil catches you plucking these hairs, you are in deep trouble.

The Devil is the father of Lies: "War is Peace," "The Clean Water Act," "Liberating the Iraqi People," "the Wisdom of the

Marketplace," "Free Society," "Competitive in the Global Economy," "Equal Opportunity," "Our Friend the Atom," "Progress is Our Most Important Product," "With Liberty and Justice for All," "Be All You Can Be," "No Child Left Behind," "It's the Real Thing."

One key unlocks all the cells of the self-imposed prison. This is the realization that the human being is not mere matter. The whole human being is body, soul, and spirit united. The Children have come to remind us in full consciousness of our spiritual nature, the true nature we have all but forgotten. But dawn is breaking.

Can we even imagine what courage, what compassion the Children of the Future bear as they come through the gateways of life into America or China or Africa? What if they should lose their way? What if they forget who they are? Just like green grass cracking the clods, children have tremendous spiritual resilience and life forces to grow against all odds and obstacles blocking the way.

Devoted teachers and well-meaning parents all across the land want to do everything within their power to help children realize their potential. But they are hindered, unable to speak of the most essential thing—the whole child as body, soul, and spirit. These are not empty words. These are living powers.

Paradoxically, in the "land of the free" the uniformity and regimentation of the educational system is blind to the true nature of children. Standardized curricula, fill-in-the-bubble tests, narrowly defined goals, and predetermined outcomes act like the frog stopping the flowing fountain, like the mouse nibbling on the roots of the Tree of Life. Words shift their shape when the "No Child Left Behind" platitude is used by a dragon for its own purposes. When children all around become anxious, pale, and burdened by sclerotic adult demands, only the Child of Good Fortune, the Spirit of Childhood can free them.

In a lightning stroke of intuition, we discover the shining ideal of the *free human being*—the Archetype of our Humanity in body, soul, and spirit. In that light we become inspired to transform education. The healing liberation that we seek in education ignites a chain reaction shift of consciousness that affects how we think about everything: health, diet, the environment, social synergy, brotherhood-sisterhood among peoples, setting humane economic and political priorities, encouraging a flowering of creativity in the arts and sciences, celebrating diversity, and discovering ourselves in our radiant humanity.

Nelson Mandela, for one, stripped of all material possessions, deprived of movement, consigned to back-breaking labor, physically and psychically punished, broke through:

> Our deepest fear is not that we are inadequate. Our deepest fear is that we are powerful beyond measure. It is our light, not our darkness, that most frightens us. We ask ourselves, 'Who am I to be brilliant, gorgeous, talented, fabulous?' Actually, who are you not to be? You are born to make manifest the glory of God that is within you. It's not just in some of us. It's in everyone. And as we let our own light shine, we unconsciously give other people permission to do the same. As we're liberated from our own fear, our presence automatically liberates others.

In this spirit of liberation we understand that we must have courage to stand boldly for the individual human spirit and the Spirit of Humanity. Rudolf Steiner, speaking of education, prophetically observed, "We have to turn the rudder 180 degrees."

> Human being, you yourself—
>   knowing, feeling, and willing—
> You are the riddle of the world.
> What in the world is concealed
> Grows manifest in you.
> It becomes light in your spirit,
> It becomes warmth in your soul.
> Your breathing welds your body's life
> To worlds of soul and realms of spirit.
> It leads you into the world of matter
> That you may find your humanity,
> And that you lose not yourself on the way,
> It guides you into spirit.

Spirit is the light of our renewal. As we lift our thoughts toward the Children of the Future preparing to take up their earthly tasks, we see the seed forces of their spiritual gifts. They are formed by and endowed with the creative forces of the universe, and I see them this way: The Child of the Future consciously bears the spiritual archetype of the human being. Into this form of forms, the elements and the mineral kingdom, coalesce the physical vessel of the body—the vehicle of earthly life. Matter, mother, Mater fills the form with earthly substance in harmonious proportion as the embryo recapitulates the age-old pattern of the species. The self-renewing physical body is a cosmic gift received into the Holy Child.

The human being is intimately related in body and soul with the plants through the breath. Breath that draws from the forming forces of the etheric world, which have lifted the plants to life and light through rhythmic transformation of dead mineral substance (earth). All medicinal plants, all fruit-bearing plants, the trees, the seed-bearing grains, all flowers wild and tame, all cultivated vegetables in root, stalk, leaf, and flower, all that is green and growing share their secrets and substance with the human being united in the kingdom of life. The Holy Child receives the gift of Life.

We share the world with the animal kingdom whose beauty, wise instincts, mobility, diversity, soul-full sentience reveal the realm of perceptive inwardness. This *astral* chain of being climbs from protozoan, to barnacle, to butterfly, to serpent, to ox, to eagle, and lion in all the boundless Imagination of Divine Creation. The timeless wisdom of the Animal Spirits is laid at the feet of the Holy Child from all quarters of the zodiac.

Within these sheathes of the physical body, the etheric body, and the astral body, the self-conscious human "I" wakes. "Let there be light." The radiant fire of the Spirit illumines the path of the Holy Child.

Active, wisdom-filled forces of the twelve senses are bestowed upon the awakening "I": the will senses of touch, well-being, movement, balance; the feeling senses of taste, smell, sight, and warmth; and the cognitive senses of hearing, thought, word, and ego. Through the portals of the senses the cosmos reveals itself to the opening soul of the Holy Child.

The Child is endowed with fiery mobility of will, the spectrum of weaving feeling, the clear light of thinking. These capacities will be used in accordance with the child's initiative and energy, love of beauty, insight and creativity. The Child receives these treasures with the generous, future-bearing impulse to use them in the service of humanity.

The universe of archetypal forms, of mathematics, of geometry, of sculpture, of architecture is offered to the Child in a spirit of creative play.

The Logos, the creative power of the Word, the gift of language, and intuitive cognition illumine the Child's consciousness. The Child cherishes these gifts with Memory, Imagination, and Meaning in profound reverence and gratitude.

The blessings of music suffuse the Child's soul with the harmony of the spheres, the angelic choirs, the resounding tones of the planets, rippling rhythms and rivers of life, and fountains of melodies.

Rainbow colors flood soul space with Beauty in all the glorious hues and harmonies of light and darkness. The Child grasps the glorious spectrum with creative delight.

Love for humanity streams into and radiates from the heart of the Child. The sister-brotherhood of the human family fires the will to serve, to work for the benefit of all, to see God in Everyman, and everywhere "To see His Name engraved in stone, and plant and beast." The Child embraces the Community of Life.

So the blessings of the world stream in upon the Child who receives them in gratitude, reverence, and freedom. So may we receive, recognize, and love the Child entrusted to our care.

❧

TO THE CHILDREN OF THE FUTURE

A child walks toward us,
A mission in her eyes,
"To be born,
I made a vow
To awake and rise,
To stand upright
Upon the ground
And speak the living word,
To keep vigil through the night
Till stars' harmony be heard,
To explore the earthly kingdoms
Of stone and plant and beast,
By clear thought to behold
The greatest in the least,
To transform clay, wood, iron, and rock
With understanding hands,
To embrace the joys and sorrows
Of my fellow Man.

If you would help me reach my goal,
Answer the question of my soul,
That I may wake, become, arise,
Tell me now, who am I?"

— — —

I alone can answer
The question that you pose,
As surely as the sunlight
Fulfills the yearning rose.

Here, now, I have come home
To form the self I will become,
And reap a harvest of ripening seeds
Joyfully sown as childhood's deeds.

United in beauty, thought, and will
We resolve to build a school
Where the wide world all
Awakes within our souls.

Here we will traverse
The depths and widths of space
To find the moving balance
Of self-sustaining grace.

Here lift dead letters to the light,
That sage and poet again are heard,
Reborn in imagination's sight
Freeing the living word.

Here traverse the rainbow bridge,
The "suffering and deeds of light,"
Till our souls are refreshed, renewed
Through colors' healing might.

Here lift heart and voice to tones,
To stretch our souls so far,
That music inspires both breath and bone
With the harmony of the stars.

Here forge new tools to our use,
Touch the language of form,
Unseal the wisdom of the will
Where intuition's born.

Here unite thought's clarity
With heart's knowing sight
To behold the tree in the seed,
The levity in light.

Here care for humble earth,
Laboring our own rebirth,
Work for good, share our gifts,
By our deeds the fallen lift,
Extend hands full of humanity,
Our brother, our sister, ourselves set free.

Here is the school
We will build
Of light and love and will,
Formed of earth
To be a home
For the waking soul.

❧

EPILOGUE

By THE CALENDAR IT has been a year and a half since my cancer surgery, and a year since my therapeutic journey to the clinics in Switzerland. By my internal clock and some trick of the imagination, the time that has passed has been both an eternity and only an instant. A status report is in order.

My ever-vigilant neuro-oncologist, Dr. Weaver, monitors my status with periodic MRIs, occasional PT scans, and a thalium scan. There has been a resurgence of the cancer at the site where it first occurred eighteen months ago. This time the resurgent tumor was discovered quickly and surgically removed for the second time. There is a five-inch seam across my fashionably bald head. Perhaps a zipper should be installed in case it comes again. Radiation treatment is long past. One radiation series is a lifetime dose. A time released chemotherapy chip has been implanted in response to this recurrence. I feel healthy and hopeful and very much alive.

Faithfully, I continue to do my therapeutic eurythmy exercises five times a week, about twenty minutes a day. I am convinced that the harmony of my body; my inner, and outer balance in thinking, feeling, and willing; my experience of healing, wholeness, and well-being are supported by these archetypal energies and gestures.

Faithfully, I continue my Iscador (mistletoe extract) injections, three times per week as long as there is any possibility of cancer recurring. My immune system is fully operational. I have more vitality and enthusiasm for life than I have had for years. Taking naps makes a virtue of necessity. Oh, well. Again, let me underscore the importance of Iscador. German and Swiss studies have researched its virtues and effects to the extent that it is now prescribed for sixty percent of German medical patients, both allopathic and anthroposophic, seeking cancer treatment therapy.

I have continued the oil dispersion hydrotherapy with what I can only call revelatory success. The transformations stimulated by these oil baths have been deeply personal and liberating. I have come a ways and have a ways to go in resolving locked places in body, soul, and spirit that can only be transformed in the deep places of the heart. That the changes are real will never be measured by EEGs or blood counts. "By their fruits, ye shall know them" in a freeing of energy long held hostage.

Quite by chance (how can I still be saying that?), I was placed in the center of thirty singing bowls, gongs, and Andean whistles and was played upon in a transport of amazement and joy. I had a powerful experience of the *Healing Power of Sound*, the title of a book by Mitchel Gaynor, M.D. Since then, I have made it a ritual to ring a singing bowl most mornings and send my thoughts, my loving intentions, to those who are making this challenging journey toward healing with me. The purity of the bowl's reverberating overtones and undertones center me and expand my soul. The ringing, singing bowl reminds me of the harmony and wholeness of the human being and the celestial harmonies of the stars from which we come and to which we return.

Healing guides continue to work on my behalf.

The Medicine Wheel has been lovingly reactivated to see me through the next stages of my transformation.

❧

Always the question lingers: who am I to be among the fortunate few to have faced glioblastoma multiforme phase IV cancer, not once but twice, and lived to tell the tale? How is this possible? By the grace of God. Meanwhile, place your bets, and ask me again in a few years. I trust I'll be around.

For now let us take to heart the words of Rudolf Steiner:

> Let us eradicate from the soul all fear and terror of
> what comes to meet us out of the future.
> Let us acquire serenity in all feelings and sensations
> about the future.
> Let us look forward with absolute equanimity to
> everything that may come
> and let us think only that whatever comes is given to us
> by a world direction full of wisdom.
> It is part of what we must learn in this age, namely, to
> live out of pure trust
> without any security in existence, trusting in the ever
> present help of the spiritual
> world. Truly nothing else will do if our courage is not
> to fail. Let us discipline
> our will and let us seek that awakening from within
> ourselves every morning and every evening.

The recent passing of a friend after eight years of cancer has brought these words back again, illumined by the intensity of shared experience. I take them to heart. This friend, more than anyone else I know, lived with death. She knew fear first-hand. But her love for life was stronger—love for her husband, for her extended family, for food and festivals, for her birds, for strays, for wild creatures, for art, for nature, for dancing, for Anthroposophy, for community, for good causes, for lost causes, for those in need. Her eight-year farewell was a death-defying, high-wire drama, a daily lesson in courage, and a triumph of the will.

Having so much time to prepare for her own death, she had assembled a care package of words and images with characteristically irreverent humor. One particular card shows mourners assembled for a funeral. A man props himself up inside his padded casket saying, "I'd just like to thank you all for coming and apologize for, once again, misjudging the severity of my illness."

Let the cosmic levity of love and laughter lighten and lift her. Casting off her bodily burden, she is free! She can visit whenever we call. Like a monarch, queen of light and air, she already tastes the honey of sorrow transformed to beauty, meaning, music, purpose, and light.

This karmic connection and others in the Medicine Wheel of our compassion are much more than memories. They are presences and helpers, "ancestors" and guides. They are a spiritual wellspring for us as our loving thoughts are spiritual bread for them. Through them I have learned that I have been held by grace and friends—living and dead—in a circle of extraordinary love, care and prayer. This has restored my life to balance and joy. For me the "meaning" of my bout with cancer has been to learn through others to love life more deeply.

Working with cancer is an initiation path that many of us will walk with those we love. "Be not afraid," on our journey. "I will fear no evil, for Thou art with me." It may be that the course of life includes painful fear and anger, a descent, the Dark Night of the Soul. So be it. It is true that isolation and "entombment" in the cancer ward are steps of grace that lead to dying, to death and to awakening to Self. These stages of transformation are not hollow abstractions. We can depend upon the refiner's fire to purge the dross of doubt, despair, and fear. In cancer's crucible, healing forces are mobilized that will drive away isolation, loneliness, and cold. Eye to eye and I to I, we take each other's hands and say simply, purely, truly: "I love you," now and forever, come what may. Warmth of love brings healing from all directions. The temporal body falls away as ash. The golden wisdom of the heart remains. Here we find the "Peace that passes all understanding." This Peace is built on the unshakable foundation of love.

∞

As we part, here at the edge of Death Valley, I feel like an old prospector handing over a weather-stained chart. "You take this map, sonny. Where I'm goin' I won't be needin' it no more. But while you're here on the earthly plane, I want you to know there is water, the *water of life*, deep down, right here. Yonder, atop

Solomon's Knob, is the Mother Lode—pay dirt, pure gold, the sun's tears. The way is steep. Just keep putting one foot in front of the other. Up on top you can see forever. Good-bye, God bless, and good luck!"

Meanwhile, my lift-off has been postponed till further notice. It's a blessing, giving me more time to prepare for my journey to Holy Jerusalem. It's a long way, but I intend to travel light.